ON SOUL
and
CONSCIENCE

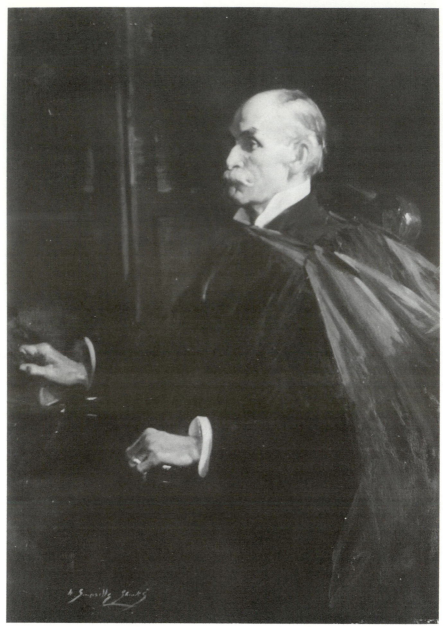

1 John Glaister Sr, fourth Regius Professor of Medical Jurisprudence and Forensic Medicine (GUA)

on Soul and Conscience

the Medical Expert and Crime

M Anne Crowther and
Brenda White

150 Years of Forensic Medicine in Glasgow

ABERDEEN UNIVERSITY PRESS

First published 1988
Aberdeen University Press
A member of the Pergamon Group

© M Anne Crowther and Brenda M White 1988

British Library Cataloguing in Publication Data

Crowther, M. Anne
  On soul and conscience.
  1. Scotland. Strathclyde Region. Glasgow.
  Forensic medicine, 1839-1989
  I. Title   II. White, Brenda M.
  614′.1′0941443

ISBN 0 08 036406 3
ISBN 0 08 036407 1 Pbk

PRINTED IN GREAT BRITAIN
THE UNIVERSITY PRESS
ABERDEEN

FOR
JOHN CROWTHER AND JOHN WHITE
TWO PATIENT MEN

Contents

Illustrations

Regius Professors of Forensic Medicine at the University of Glasgow

Robert Cowan	1839-1841
Harry Rainy	1841-1872
Pierce Adolphus Simpson	1872-1898
John Glaister, Sr	1898-1931
John Glaister, Jr	1931-1962
Gilbert Forbes	1964-1974
William Arthur Harland	1974-1985
Alan Albert Watson	1985-

Preface

'The *Justices*, with us, do never accept of the single *Testimonies* of Physicians and Chirurgeons, but oblige them to depone or declare upon *oath* ... and for the same cause the *Justices* do reject *Testificats* subscribed by them, unless bearing upon *Soul* and *Conscience*.' (Sir Alexander Seton, 1699)

In a Scottish murder trial, when the medical expert gives his evidence, the jury hears him read out a detailed report of the work he has done, and of his findings. In an English court, the medical witness would refer to notes made at the time 'to refresh his memory'; but the Scottish report is a formal piece of evidence, produced along with the gun or the bloodstained knife as an exhibit; and its author will be questioned on it by prosecution and defence. The doctor has signed it under the words 'on soul and conscience', the form of oath used by his profession since the seventeenth century: indeed, if he fails to use this phrase he may be fined 'one hundred merks Scots', though as this penalty has long fallen into disuse, the court might have difficulty translating it into current coin.

Acknowledgments

The research for this book was largely financed by a generous grant from the Wellcome Trust, which has done so much to encourage medical history in Scotland. We were also assisted at an early stage by a travel grant from the Carnegie Trust, which we gratefully acknowledge.

We were first introduced to the project by Michael Moss and Derek Dow, archivists and entrepreneurs: our thanks to them, and to Lesley Richmond for their help and advice in Glasgow University Archives.

We have been most fortunate in being able to draw on a large number of personal papers, press-cuttings and medical reports preserved by Professor John Glaister Jr, and now in the care of Dr David McLay, Chief Medical Officer to the Strathclyde Police. Dr McLay most generously allowed us to retain the papers while writing this book, and also assisted us with his knowledge of the history of the Glasgow police surgeons.

We are also grateful to the following librarians and archivists in Glasgow: Mr Andrew Rogers and Mr Laurence Bebbington of the library of the Royal College of Physicians and Surgeons of Glasgow; the staff of Glasgow University library, especially Trevor Graham, who prepared the photographs, and Jean Robertson; Mr Joe Fisher and the staff of the Glasgow Room at the Mitchell library; the archivists of the Strathclyde Regional archives; the librarians of the Royal Faculty of Procurators in Glasgow; and Mr W G Doig of the *Glasgow Herald* picture library.

In Edinburgh, the staff of the Scottish Record Office, particularly Mr George Barbour, Mr Bruno Longmore, and Mr Peter Vasey, were extremely helpful, and located uncatalogued records for us. We also received valuable assistance from the staff of Edinburgh University Library, and from Mrs M B Paton of the Advocates Library.

Our research into the role of the Crown Office was much aided by Mr Andrew Normand, formerly of the Crown Office, and now Procurator Fiscal for Airdrie, and Mr A D Vannet of the Crown Office. Mr Eric Cumming, Depute Clerk to the Judiciary, and Mr W G O'Hara of the High Court, Glasgow, assisted our investigations into Scottish legal procedures.

Dr William Rodger, Director of the Strathclyde Police Forensic Laboratory, and Dr James Thorpe of the University of Strathclyde, gave us much helpful information on the background and current work of forensic scientists in

Glasgow. We are also grateful to Professor John Lenihan for his friendly assistance with the complexities of activation analysis.

We should like to thank the following for their courtesy in assisting us with personal information: Mrs Morag Arthur, (née Glaister); Dr Andrew Allison; Mr Richard Beavers; Professor Donald Campbell; Sir David Cuthbertson; Mr Jack House; Mr Bill Knox; Dr Walter Spilg; Dr Wright Thomson; and Dr John Wallace.

At the beginning of our work, we were able to benefit from discussion with the sixth and seventh Regius Professors of Forensic Medicine, the late Gilbert Forbes, and the late Arthur Harland.

We are grateful to the Scottish Record Office, the Crown Office, and Strath-clyde Regional Archives, for permission to quote from unpublished material, and to the *Glasgow Herald* for permission to reproduce photographs from their archives.

To the present staff of the department of Forensic Medicine and Science of the University of Glasgow, we owe a special debt. All staff, secretarial, technical and academic, bore with our interruptions into their busy lives, and answered our questions with great patience. Without their aid, this project would have been impossible. In this collective acknowledgment, however, we must single out Alan Watson, eighth Regius Professor of Forensic Medicine, and Hamilton Smith, Professor of Toxicology, for their unfailing support.

This book was written by two social historians, who take responsibility for any errors within it. Although we have greatly appreciated the advice of medical, legal and scientific experts, the arguments which follow are our own.

Glossary

The text refers to Scottish legal terms which may be unfamiliar.

culpable homicide	A criminal charge similar to the English charge of manslaughter
Lord Advocate	the chief law officer in Scotland, appointed by the government of the day.
panel or pannell	the accused person
precognitions	statements of witnesses and others submitted to the Procurator Fiscal, on the basis of which he may decide to prosecute. The defence may also precognose witnesses.
Procurators Fiscal	Lawyers appointed by the Lord Advocate, with the duty of initiating prosecutions: they combine the functions of coroner and public prosecutor
productions	any objects, documents, etc produced in court ('exhibits' in English courts)

Abbreviations

ARCCG	*Annual Report of the Chief Constable of Glasgow*
DPH	Diploma in Public Health
BMJ	*British Medical Journal*
Ed.Med.Surg.Jnl.	*Edinburgh Medical and Surgical Journal*
EMJ	*Edinburgh Medical Journal*
EUL	Edinburgh University Library, Special Collections
GET	*Glasgow Evening Times*
GH	*Glasgow Herald*
GMC	General Medical Council
GMJ	*Glasgow Medical Journal*
GP	Glaister papers, (see bibliography)
GRI	Glasgow Royal Infirmary
GUA	Glasgow University Archives
GUL	Glasgow University Library
HMSO	His (Her) Majesty's Stationery Office
Jnl.Clin.Pathol.	*Journal of Clinical Pathology.*
Jnl.Forensic Sci.Soc.	*Journal of the Forensic Science Society*
Med.Hist.	*Medical History*
Med.Sci.Law	*Medicine, Science and the Law*
MOH	Medical Officer of Health
NHS	National Health Service
PP	British Parliamentary Papers
PRO	Public Record Office, London
RCPS	Library of the Royal College of Physicians and Surgeons of Glasgow
Scot.Med.Jnl.	*Scottish Medical Journal*
SRA	Strathclyde Regional Archives, Glasgow
SRO	Scottish Record Office, Edinburgh
Trans.Med.Leg.Soc.	*Transactions of the Medico-Legal Society*
Wellcome	Wellcome Library, London

Introduction

This is a description, from a particular angle, of New Year's Day in Glasgow a few years ago.

In the city, the Hogmanay celebrations were energetic, and the police had a busy night. Since it is a public holiday, shops and offices are closed: the University, also, has thriftily turned off the heating in most buildings, and only the most determined scholar would look for refuge there. Lights are burning, however, in 8 University Gardens. This elegant house, part of an imposing Victorian terrace, was built in 1895 for Joseph Coats, Professor of Pathology, and once witnessed elaborate dinner-parties attended by some of the most eminent medical men of the time. Now, having been converted into the department of forensic medicine in 1955, it is put to uses which its architect never expected. The room where Lord Lister dined is now the office of the Regius Professor of Forensic Medicine; the large living room on the ground floor is a library and study for graduate students; the maids' room is full of microcomputers; other domestic offices are filled by the machines for toxicological analysis.

Like their clinical colleagues in the neighbouring Western Infirmary, the forensic pathologists in the department are busy at Hogmanay, and they are expected to be at the disposal of the police throughout this season. In the city mortuary, the pathologists examine some of the citizens of Glasgow for whom the revels have ended abruptly: afterwards, samples of human tissue may be taken to the university laboratory to be prepared for examination under the microscope. Later, the toxicologists in the department will test any samples sent to them for drugs and alcohol.

Shortly before this book was completed, the department regretfully left the ornate plasterwork and carved wood of University Gardens, and moved into a new building with purpose-built laboratories. The size and expense of these is ample evidence of the service offered to the West of Scotland. The University is now one of several independent units in a forensic service which includes the large laboratories of the Strathclyde Police, and the work of hospital pathologists and other experts. All these have their own histories, but as the university was the starting point of much of this enterprise, we will trace its origins from here.

The first professor of medical jurisprudence and medical police was

1

appointed by the Crown in 1839, and the department celebrates its 150th anniversary in 1989. Robert Cowan, the first regius professor, was the second such appointment in Britain: the University of Edinburgh had received a similar regius chair in 1807, but Glasgow has proved to be the largest and most durable of the Scottish departments. In the university world nothing is certain, but in Glasgow the Crown has begun to subsidise the work of the forensic pathologists, and so has relieved the university of some of the financial pressure which has weakened forensic medicine elsewhere.

The history of this department is of more than local interest. The medical expert now has a respected place in British courts of law, but it has taken him a long time to win it. Forensic medicine in Glasgow, practised both in the university and by other doctors in the city, has had an important place in this process. Nineteenth-century England produced several distinguished medical experts, but they flourished mainly as individuals, without leaving a permanent establishment behind them. Scotland, where forensic medicine was embedded in the medical schools, paid far more attention to the subject, and the Scottish legal system also encouraged the rise of the medical expert. Scottish expertise provoked frequent envious comments south of the border, and the remark of Lord Trenchard in 1934, while unsuccessfully trying to create a medico-legal institute in London, may stand as one of many: 'We are a long way behind Scotland and foreign countries.'[1]

For many centuries, doctors have been summoned into court to advise the law on matters where they are believed to have special skill. At various times in history they have been asked to look for the signs of witchcraft; to make astrological comments; to detect poison in the bodies of men and animals; to test for virginity and for impotence.[2] The demands made on medical witnesses have changed as society changes, though the need to find out the cause of death in doubtful cases has been one of the most long-standing reasons why the doctors' evidence has been required.

In Britain, the doctors have had a special position in court since the seventeenth century. By that time, under English and Scots law, witnesses were not allowed to give opinions, but were required to speak only of facts; the doctors, however, as 'expert' witnesses, could give an opinion on events which they had not actually seen, to speculate, for example, on the cause of death. Their evidence might be drawn from an autopsy on the body, though such post-mortem examinations were not common in Britain until the eighteenth century, much later than their use on the Continent.[3]

The most publicised activity of forensic medicine is in the detection of causes of death, particularly homicide, but forensic medicine still implies much more than this. Its older name of 'medical jurisprudence', reveals its origins in the needs of the law, rather than as a branch of the healing arts. Essentially, it places medical knowledge at the service of the law for many purposes: deciding compensation for injury; investigating fatal accidents and injuries at work; advising on the mental state of those accused of crimes or who die leaving disputed wills; examining the victims of rape and other assaults; checking the health of applicants for life insurance policies, and so on. Like all branches of medicine, forensic medicine has become specialised. At the beginning of the twentieth century, the professors of medical jurisprudence had to deal with every aspect of forensic science from ballistics to psychiatry, but as new and complicated techniques were developed, expertise was divided between doctors, scientists and technicians. The Glasgow department now contains scientists and lawyers as well as pathologists: the division of responsibility within it, and the division of labour with other laboratories in the city, are the result of this historical expansion of the forensic sciences.

The history of medicine often gives a misleading impression of progress from one success to another: in fact, the path has usually been full of wrong turnings and difficult places. Forensic medicine is no exception, for although society takes the medical expert for granted, and assumes he will always appear when necessary, forensic medicine has been less secure than most other branches of medicine. With the exception of a few professional police surgeons, the legal system has always called in medical experts as casual labour. The work of police surgeons, however, has tended to move away from forensic pathology, as their time becomes more occupied with clinical cases such as rape and assault. Forensic scientists may find employment in police or government laboratories, but forensic pathologists must look for a career either in the hospitals or the universities, because their criminal work will not bring in a regular income. National Health Service hospitals and the universities may then feel that they are subsidising a public service which ought to be financed by the Crown: ever since the department began, the cost of maintaining forensic medicine has been disputed within Glasgow University.

There are relatively few forensic pathologists, and few career openings; consequently, most English universities see little point in making forensic medicine a compulsory part of their examination syllabus. Several universities have supported distinguished professors of forensic medicine, but, faced with the need for economies, are abolishing these posts when their holders retire. Where will the next generation of forensic specialists come from?

Forensic medicine was able to survive in Scottish universities because, unlike the English practice, it was a compulsory part of the examinations in both law and medicine. The nineteenth-century arguments which made forensic medicine compulsory for students in Edinburgh and in Glasgow were as follows: although very few doctors could make their living by forensic medicine, most were at some time called to give evidence in court, and training in forensic medicine would assist them. Also, general practitioners were often the first to encounter suspicious circumstances, and should know when to ask for expert advice. Lawyers, too, it was said, needed training in forensic medicine so that advocates could understand the use of medical evidence in court: after 1856, a knowledge of medical jurisprudence was compulsory for membership of the Faculty of Advocates.[4] These arguments are still used today, but they were not the only reason for appointing professors of the subject in nineteenth-century Scottish universities. Forensic medicine was always bracketed with public health, and in the University of Glasgow it did not stand alone until the 1920s. Teaching forensic medicine and public health together under the single title of 'Medical Police' was a Continental practice, and was one of the many links formed between Scotland and Europe in the age of the Enlightenment. The first two chapters of this book spend some time discussing the relationship between forensic medicine and public health, and if this seems far removed from the use of medicine in criminal detection today, it should be remembered that Scottish universities were prepared to support several distinguished professors of forensic medicine precisely because these men could teach the theory of sewers and ventilation as well as how to detect a murder. This eminently practical combination of skills helped to keep forensic medicine alive in Scottish medical education.

At the end of its first 150 years, we follow the history of the Glasgow department from its original connection with the public health movement, through the heroic age of the medical detectives, to the more specialised teamwork and complex research of the present day. The department has existed for three purposes: teaching, research, and providing expert services to the police and courts of law. Sometimes one or other of these activities has predominated: keeping a balance between them is difficult. The first three regius professors rarely appeared in court, but the five appointed since 1898 have been constantly in the public eye through the reporting of trials in the local and national press. The days are gone when the local newspapers (far more numerous than at present), sent shorthand reporters to give an almost verbatim account of the professor's evidence, but the forensic pathologists still have to contend with a higher degree of public interest in their work than most of their medical colleagues experience. A problem in diagnosis, rather than being left to quiet discussion behind hospital walls, may be followed by the excited headline 'TOP DOCS BAFFLED!'

Away from the publicity were the less spectacular but essential functions of teaching and research. These ensured that the department could survive the retirement of the brilliant individualists. To that extent it has, so far, been untypical of the fortunes of forensic medicine in the British university system, for the nation expects total efficiency from the forensic services, but is not always prepared to pay for it.

CHAPTER ONE

Early Years: 1839-1898

In 1839 the University of Glasgow occupied a modest group of buildings around a courtyard in the High Street. Its once convenient central site had been overwhelmed by the growth of the city, and was now surrounded by reeking and overcrowded tenements, amongst which the ancient institution sat in grimy dignity. On the 15 July, the Principal, the Reverend Dr Duncan Macfarlan, opened his morning newspaper and gleaned from its columns that his university had acquired two new regius professors, one for the theory of physic, and the other for medical jurisprudence.[1] The Principal was enraged. Regius professors were chosen by the Crown—in practice, the government of the day—and the Principal and Senate of the university had no control over their appointment.[2] Even if the Principal had wanted two more professors, which he did not, he would not have been pleased, for Lord Melbourne's Whig government was in power, and the Principal and most of the Senate were staunch Tories. The new professors would, as a result of Crown patronage, inevitably be Whigs.

The Principal decided to ignore the government's action. When Senate met on 7 August, it created a lectureship in medical jurisprudence instead of the chair, and immediately elected Allan Burns, son of the professor of surgery, to fill it.[3] The Clerk of Senate, however, was legally obliged to produce the warrants, signed by Queen Victoria, appointing Robert Cowan as professor of medical jurisprudence and forensic medicine, and Andrew Buchanan as professor of the theory of physic. The Principal appealed against the two appointments to the Rector, Sir James Graham, a prominent Tory, but nothing could be done to prevent them. Under the circumstances, Allan Burns declined the lectureship. The Principal had then to acknowledge these unwelcome professors, knowing, however, that they could be kept at arm's length. The small, oligarchic group of professors who made up the College Faculty controlled the endowments of the university, and elected new members to their own ranks whenever a chair fell vacant. The regius professors were not members of the Faculty, and had no part in the important financial decisions of the university.

In this contentious fashion, the first professor of forensic medicine was imposed on the University of Glasgow. Political rather than academic considerations were uppermost, but the study of forensic medicine could not be

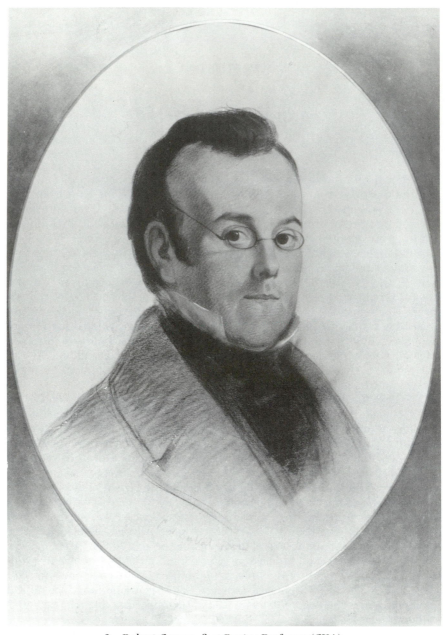

2   Robert Cowan, first Regius Professor (GUA)

separated from politics. To understand why the subject aroused such passions, it is necessary to go back to Edinburgh at the beginning of the nineteenth century, and the foundation of the first British chair in medical jurisprudence.

From 1807 until the early 1830s, the University of Edinburgh was the only medical school in Britain to give systematic instruction in forensic medicine. This contrasted with almost total apathy towards the subject in England. In 1831 the Society of Apothecaries in London required that all students seeking its licence attend a course of lectures in forensic medicine, and some of the London hospitals responded by appointing lecturers in the subject, but the Society's standards were not rigorous,[4] and, since the students were not examined in forensic medicine, they did not take it very seriously. In Edinburgh, on the other hand, medical jurisprudence, which was already a popular subject, became a compulsory part of the medical examinations in 1833. Glasgow, slow to follow Edinburgh's example, nevertheless in 1839 introduced forensic medicine as a compulsory part of the medical examinations.

Why did the Scottish universities take this early interest in forensic medicine? It would be pleasing, but wrong, to argue that the medical schools of Scotland had a superior understanding of the value of forensic medicine in detecting crime. In fact, when the Edinburgh chair was founded, criminal investigation was a secondary motive. The techniques of forensic medicine, particularly in Britain, were rudimentary, and its benefits by no means obvious.[5] Doctors were usually called into court to give evidence on such matters as the cause of death and the nature of wounds; to detect poisons; to say whether a dead baby had been born alive and whether a woman had recently been delivered; to comment on legitimacy and sanity: but all of these subjects were very uncertain, and often led to disputes between medical witnesses. Two of Scotland's most distinguished expatriates of the eighteenth century, the brothers William and John Hunter, were interested in forensic questions: John Hunter with his study of gunshot wounds, and the way in which the stomach lining could be digested after death (leading to baseless suspicions of poisoning); William Hunter in a famous essay, *On the Uncertainty of the Signs of Murder, in the case of Bastard Children* (1783). Yet the Hunters' work helped rather to expose the enormous gaps in medical knowledge than to inspire confidence in medical witnesses. The chair in Edinburgh owed less to the advancement of medical knowledge than to political disputes, in which forensic medicine was secondary to the subject with which it was coupled in Scotland, 'medical police', or the study of hygiene. By the time the Glasgow chair was founded, forensic medicine was more important in its own right, but, as in Edinburgh, it was firmly associated with 'medical police'.

The eighteenth-century theory of 'medical police', had originated in Germany and spread to other parts of Europe.[6] It may be briefly defined as the use of medicine in the service of the state, both to protect the health of its subjects, and to keep them under control. Under the mercantilist ideas then current, a large and healthy population was essential to both to the state's wealth and its military power, hence the need for 'medical police'.[7] The use of the word 'police' now seems strange because of its modern association with the constabulary, but its older meaning was 'polity', or 'civil order'. Until the nineteenth century, the Scottish use of the word 'police' or 'polis' referred to all the petty government of a community, including cleansing.[8] The theory of medical police showed how medicine could serve government in many ways, but two services of particular importance were the maintenance of public health and the detection of crime.

Britain had, in contrast to many European countries, a relatively weak central government and a small bureaucracy. The 'enlightened' autocratic governments of Europe aspired towards a central administration, and did not lack advice on how to make it efficient. The most comprehensive German theory, J P Frank's massive *System of Medical Police*,[9] would have involved rigorous control over both the environment and personal hygiene. Everything which related to public health, from street cleaning to prostitution, would have been subjected to state control. Although these interventionist theories had some roots in actual practice, such as the use of quarantine during epidemics, most of them were not really workable under eighteenth-century conditions. Yet they left a legacy in European medical education, and were part of the rise of 'scientific medicine' at the end of the eighteenth century.

The Scottish interest in medical police was one of the many links between Edinburgh and the Continent at the time of the Scottish Enlightenment. By the end of the eighteenth century, the University of Edinburgh had become a famous centre of medical education, and had the only substantial law school in Scotland.[10] The upper ranks of Scottish society, usually less wealthy than their English counterparts, were debarred both by Presbyterianism and poverty from sending their sons to Oxford and Cambridge; but a period of travel and study abroad, still relatively cheap, added a desirable polish to a Scottish education. European scholars visited the Scottish universities, and Scottish intellectual life was responsive to European influences.

Medical police, however, had become a revolutionary subject by the end of the eighteenth century. The French Revolution destroyed the old medical schools of France and set up new ones based on practical observation rather than classical theory. Medical police rapidly became an interest of the revolutionary state, which saw the health of the population as essential to the success of its huge citizen army. At the same time, the battlefields provided military surgeons with greater practical experience than ever encountered in previous wars, and increased their knowledge of anatomy.[11] The new medical schools of France included many teachers whose careers had begun as army surgeons, and amongst the subjects for compulsory study, dictated by the state, was forensic medicine (*médecine légale*), which included the study of medical police. A chair of legal medicine was founded in Paris in 1795, and during the nineteenth century was occupied by some of the most distinguished figures in European forensic medicine.[12] In 1804 a chair of forensic medicine and medical police was also founded in Vienna, and study of these subjects was compulsory. In Britain, however, the French revolution provoked a great political upheaval, with radical Whigs saluting the revolutionary emphasis on liberty and the rights of the citizen, while the Tories denounced any connection with it. The study of medical police could be seen as a practical creation of the revolution. To certain radical thinkers in Britain it seemed a way of improving the efficiency of the state and serving the ends of justice: to the Tories, it was a foreign and possibly dangerous import.

The chief link between European theory and Scottish practice came through Andrew Duncan, Professor of the Institutes of Medicine at Edinburgh, who in 1795 began a series of lectures on medical jurisprudence within his main lecture course. Duncan was familiar with Continental theories of medical police, both German and French, and particularly admired the work of Frank. In 1798 he wrote a memorial to the patrons of the university, urging them to institute a chair in medical jurisprudence. Duncan saw the benefits of this subject as twofold: the first concerned forensic medicine, both for the detection of crime and settling of civil disputes, the second, 'of incomparably greater consequence', was medical police, which 'regards not merely the welfare of individuals, but the prosperity and security of nations'.[13] As the European example dictated, Duncan saw forensic medicine and public health as inseparable, though his version of medical police adapted the European theory into a less coercive form, suited to the decentralised government of Britain.[14]

Duncan's views seemed to stand little chance of success. The Town Council, which controlled university appointments, had no interest in forensic medicine, and the professors of the university always disliked additions to their own number. Professors, especially in medicine, received much of their income from student fees, and the appointment of extra professors meant that fees were spread more thinly. The Crown also had the power to create a new chair, but the Dundas family had for several decades exercised Scottish patronage in the Tory interest: Duncan was a well-known Whig, and medical police a radical notion. The Edinburgh Senate rejected the proposed chair, as bringing no dignity or prosperity to the university.[15]

The Edinburgh Whigs, lacking political power, nevertheless included some of the most distinguished figures in Scottish intellectual life. The young radicals who founded and wrote for the *Edinburgh Review* included a number of able lawyers who were determined to reform the Scottish legal system. Reform was a complex affair, for Scottish law was encumbered by antique regulations. Amongst other changes, the Whigs proposed to introduce juries in civil cases, and to end the judges' power of selecting the jurymen in criminal cases.

The Edinburgh Whigs, prompted by Duncan, included the study of medical police as part of their scheme for legal reform. Duncan not only contributed to the *Edinburgh Review*, but founded the *Edinburgh Medical and Surgical Journal*, one of the most respected nineteenth-century medical periodicals. It did not try to separate medicine from politics: its first volume, published in 1805, carried a long and respectful review of two weighty French treatises on medical police, one by Paul Mahon, the professor of legal medicine in Paris.[16] The reviewer noted approvingly that Mahon saw forensic medicine as a process of 'natural justice'—a phrase especially irritating to Tories because of its connection with radical writers like William Godwin.

Duncan's chance came in 1806 during the brief Whig government known as the 'Ministry of all the Talents'. He had impressed his ideas upon his close friend, Henry Erskine, who became Lord Advocate under the Whig administration, and Erskine persuaded the government to establish a chair of 'Medical Jurisprudence and Medical Police' in Edinburgh. The medical faculty refused to receive the new chair, and it stayed in the faculty of law until 1825: in 1833 it became an established part of the medical curriculum. Erskine used the words of Duncan's memorial to justify the social usefulness of medical jurisprudence, stressing the protection of property as much as the detection of violent crime. In the fashion of contemporary politics, mixing intellectual commitment with self-interest, Duncan ensured that the man appointed to the new chair in 1807 was his own son, Andrew Duncan Jr.

Although the Tories were soon returned to office, and there was complaint in Parliament that the new chair was a piece of political provocation,[17] it was not discontinued when its first occupant resigned for a more prestigious chair (though he was replaced by a Tory professor). In the 1820s, a second Tory appointment, Robert Christison, made the chair famous: he not only took part in several notorious cases, such as that of Burke and Hare, but conducted much original research into violent deaths and wrote the first major work on toxicology in English. Christison approached the subject differently from the Duncans, and shifted the balance of the teaching away from public health towards forensic medicine, but his successors continued to teach both with varying emphases according to their own interests. Christison played a crucial part in showing that forensic medicine was a respectable academic subject, and successfully persuaded the medical faculty in Edinburgh to accept it, but in a Scottish medical education, forensic medicine and public health were still inseparable subjects.

By the time Glasgow received its own regius chair in 1839, the scientific side of forensic medicine had made modest progress, though the most applauded discovery, Marsh's test for arsenic, was made only in 1836.[18] The success of men like Christison depended on careful post-mortem examinations, close observation and common sense rather than technical developments. The main message of British forensic medicine, as practised by Christison and English experts like Alfred Swaine Taylor, was that medical men should be cautious in the witness box, and not risk public contempt by pretending to more knowledge than they possessed.

The companion subject of medical police seemed less revolutionary after the ending of the French wars, but was still associated with political groups who supported social reform. In Glasgow, as in Edinburgh, the question of medical police was important in the foundation of a chair. In 1826 a Royal Commission was appointed to investigate the antiquated government of the

Scottish Universities: it visited Glasgow the following year, and the question of a chair in medical jurisprudence was raised. Only John Burns, the professor of surgery, was prepared to give any support to forensic medicine, since he thought Glasgow lagged behind Edinburgh:

> It is certainly of very considerable importance too, with a view to the public appearance of medical men, when they are examined; it is of importance to the life, death, and character of the panel, which may sometimes depend on their judgment. The guilty may be acquitted and the innocent convicted by erroneous opinions.[19]

In common with general thinking on universities at that time,[20] Burns did not regard a new chair as a way of advancing knowledge, but purely as an enhancement to medical education and prestige.

The other professors of medicine in Glasgow had no time for forensic medicine. Of the eight medical professors, only three had a place on the powerful College Faculty, but all objected to subdivision of their teaching and the resulting loss of income from fees. James Jeffray, whose tenure of the chair of anatomy lasted from 1790 to 1848, was the most powerful professor in the College. He had seen several changes in the medical curriculum: early in the century, the chairs of surgery and botany had been founded, and the new professors had taken over subjects which Jeffray had previously taught himself. Having lost income in this way, Jeffray was no champion of further medical specialisation. His views on medical jurisprudence were frank: he did not think enough was known about it to fill a lecture course. Those parts of the subject which were important, he argued, were in three areas: 'injuries, which should be taken up by the professor of surgery; poisons, which should be treated of by the professor of surgery; and Child Murder, which naturally falls to the professor of midwifery.'[21] The odd notion that toxicology should be taught by the professor of surgery rather than the professor of chemistry can be explained simply by Jeffray's hostility to the current professor of chemistry, Thomas Thomson, who wanted university reform. Other professors were happy that forensic medicine should be portioned between surgery, chemistry and midwifery, thus securing their own financial interests.[22]

The chair in Edinburgh had been supported by the faculty of law, rather than the medical faculty, but this was not possible in Glasgow. The Royal Commission's report exposed the low state into which legal studies in Glasgow had fallen since the turn of the century. The professor taught mainly Roman Law. His students, few in number, were usually clerks and apprentices, who needed a certificate of attendance at one law class before they could be admitted to the Glasgow Faculty of Procurators. Anyone with higher amibitions in Scottish law went on to study in Edinburgh.[23] No real interest in medical jurisprudence could be expected here.

Reform of the Scottish universities was a question which cut across many vested interests, and until 1858, when the Universities (Scotland) Act was passed, the universities tried to avoid government interference by permitting some internal reforms, modernising their courses, and improving their examination procedures.[24] Glasgow accepted some changes in 1833, but forensic medicine, without any backing within the university, was lost to sight: instead, it put down roots in the city's extra-mural medical schools. James Armour began to teach it at the newly formed Portland Street medical school in 1826, and John Macmichan Pagan took over in 1830; George Watt began a course at the Andersonian in 1831. In the same year, the Faculty of Physicians and Surgeons of Glasgow, who frequently quarrelled with the university over the right to grant medical licenses, stipulated that attendance at a six-months' course of lectures in medical jurisprudence would be necessary for its diploma: Pagan and Armour, influential in the Faculty, sponsored this policy.[25] Since the university provided no such courses, the extra-mural lecturers would monopolise the fees.

In Glasgow, an interest in forensic medicine, for civic and legal purposes, developed outside the university. Under Scots law, the procurators fiscal had the right to summon any medical man they pleased to perform autopsies or clinical examinations. Unlike the English coroner, the fiscals had the duty both of determining cause of death and acting as public prosecutors. Coroners were elected officials of local government, often with no particular qualification for the task, whereas the fiscals were lawyers appointed by the Lord Advocate. Some fiscals regarded the selection of medical witnesses as a chance for personal patronage—perhaps as a way of increasing the income of a medical relative—but in the towns it was customary to summon a medical man with special skills. In Edinburgh, Robert Christison had ensured that the professor of medical jurisprudence would be called by the prosecution in serious cases: in Glasgow the Crown often summoned James Corkindale, who was surgeon to the town's gaol and bridewell, secretary to the local Board of Health during the first cholera epidemic, and a powerful figure both in the Royal Infirmary and the Faculty of Physicians and Surgeons. Corkindale, in his evidence to the Royal Commission, strongly advocated a chair in medical jurisprudence, and used his influence in the city administration to put pressure on the university.

In the Senate papers of 1832 there is a memorial urging the need for a 'Teacher' in medical jurisprudence: unfortunately, its provenance is now lost, but it was obviously important enough for the Senate to consider seriously whether to create a lectureship.[26] The memorial rejected the idea that a course could be cobbled together from different elements of the medical curriculum, and, after describing the advanced state of medical education on the Continent, noted:

> In the University of Edinburgh, which has always continued to be the most complete Medical School in His Majesty's Dominions, there has been a chair of Medical Jurisprudence for more than twenty five years. Of late much interest has been drawn to this subject, both from the public in general, and from the two connected Professions, Law and Medicine. This has been owing, at least in part, to the severe, tho' just animadversions, which, on many occasions, have fallen both from the Bench and Bar on the deficiency of medical practitioners, when called upon to give evidence in Courts of Law: and that in questions, when the fortunes the honour and the lives of their fellow subjects were in jeopardy.

The memorial stressed that many licensing corporations, including the Society of Apothecaries and the Royal Colleges, the Royal College of Surgeons in Edinburgh, and the Faculty of Physicians and Surgeons of Glasgow, now required attendance at lectures in medical jurisprudence—if the university did not offer these courses, students would go elsewhere:

> The students therefore cannot help themselves. A course of Medical Jurisprudence they must have; and they will go where it is to be obtained. Every kind of instruction, like an article of Manufacture, will, if in demand, be supplied somewhere; and it appears, on many accounts to be improper that the student should be forced to go without the pale of the College for any course of lectures which he requires.

Corkindale himself, who was possibly behind this memorial, obviously hoped to be offered a lectureship, and had his application printed in anticipation. It offered the support of the Lord Provost, the Town Council, Town Clerk, Trades House and several eminent members of the Scottish legal profession.[27] Significantly, there was almost no support from the medical profession for his candidacy. The Senate decided that, since no English institution apart from the Society of Apothecaries showed much regard for medical jurisprudence, it could safely be ignored in Glasgow.[28]

Although the university denied the importance of forensic medicine, civic support for it came through the claims of medical police, which were dramatically revived in 1832. As Asiatic cholera approached across the Continent, Britain, with little experience of government regulation in time of plague, had no administration to deal with it: local government bore the chief responsibility. Local Boards of Health were set up to embark on cleansing and other sanitary campaigns if they seemed desirable, but were in many parts of Britain opposed by property interests. The central issues of medical police, quarantine, cleansing, and treatment of the infected, were debated intensely but ineffectually.

The epidemic struck Scotland particularly hard: in Edinburgh and Glasgow, the populations were tightly penned within the narrow wynds, lacking the most elementary sanitation. Chadwick's sanitary report a few years later described Glasgow as being 'both in the structural arrangements and the condition of the population ... the worst of any we had seen in any part of Great Britain.'[29] Cholera afflicted Glasgow more than any other British city in 1832, with more than 3,000 deaths.[30] This experience left behind a vocal public health lobby in Scotland, leading in time to more rigorous sanitary powers for local government than in English cities.

Prominent in the Glasgow public health movement was Robert Cowan, physician and surgeon at the Royal Infirmary. He came from a well-connected family, which had for seven generations produced academic and medical men: his forebears had given land to the University. Cowan helped to found the Glasgow Statistical Society in 1835, specifically to investigate the relationship between living standards and the incidence of disease in the west of Scotland. He became particularly interested in epidemiology, and published several pamphlets on Glasgow's fever statistics. Since there was no registration of deaths, he had to collect mortality statistics himself from the Bills of Mortality and church records.[31] Cowan argued for the introduction of a medical or 'sanatory' police in addition to the constables already operating in the city.[32]

In 1837 the University of Glasgow was again subjected to the visit of a Royal Commission, since the report of 1831 had been largely abortive, and an attempt in 1836 by Melbourne's government to bring in a reform Bill for the Scottish Universities had also failed.[33] The Commission reported in 1839, and the Senate was alarmed at the prospect of another Scottish Universities Bill which would sweep away the old oligarchy. This was not the only threat. The long debate on medical registration, which led through sixteen unsuccessful Bills to the Medical Act of 1858, had revived.[34] In 1839, pro-posals to set up a system of registration based on the University of London threatened the position of the Scottish universities.[35] In a flurry of anxiety, the Glasgow Senate devised new regulations for the medical degree, although the professors still objected to any enlargement of the curriculum if it meant new professors and more competition for fees. The Royal Commission's report in 1839 recommended two new chairs in Biblical criticism and the theory of physic, and their scheme of attendance at medical classes included a term's course in medical jurisprudence. The new regulations for the medical degree, issued in April 1839, required four years of study, and included a course of 'not less than three months' in forensic medicine. The Senate hoped to avoid having extra professors imposed on it by appointing lecturers, for these would be inexpensive and within the Senate's control.

On hearing of the Senate's decision to appoint a lecturer in forensic medicine, Robert Cowan and Andrew Buchanan offered themselves as can-didates. When they learned that university nepotism had already reserved the post for Allan Burns, political influence was brought to bear. Cowan was not only a vigorous sanitarian, but an active Whig: Buchanan shared his political views. Buchanan's brother was a friend of the Glasgow MP James Oswald, who had previously introduced an unsuccessful bill to reform the University of Glasgow. Oswald wrote to Fox Maule, under-secretary to Lord Normanby, the Secretary for War in Melbourne's administration. The Whigs were at that moment under pressure in the House, and so Oswald's letter recommending that two regius chairs be established for Cowan and Buchanan, carried some urgency. He wrote:

> Now for the College chairs—Since writing you I have thought much about them, and the result of my cogitations is, that I implore you to make the appointments without delay—you are in power, and long may you remain in power, but there is no saying what may happen, and if Sir Robert Peel was in, both Chairs would be filled instanter—The Principal would take good care of that—By making the appointments immediately, all danger is put a stop to, and the liberal interest in the College greatly strengthened ... Delays are dangerous—once more I implore you to appoint.[36]

These were the manoeuvres which lay behind Principal Macfarlan's unpleasant discovery in his morning paper. The two appointments provoked an agitated correspondence in the *Lancet*, whose editor commented sternly:

> both the creation of such appointments, and the mode of electing to them, is altogether corrupt, and highly injurious to the character of our medical institutions, and to the best interests of medical students.[37]

Once calm was restored, Robert Cowan was admitted to office after a professorial trial on his Latin essay *de Medicina Forensi*.[38] The title of his chair appeared in the royal warrant as 'Medical Jurisprudence and Forensic Medicine', but Cowan styled himself 'Professor of Medical Jurisprudence and Medical Police', on the Edinburgh model, and was so described in the university calendars. No record survives of what he taught, but his name was connected mainly with the public health movement, and he seems to have had little interest in criminal investigation. In 1840 he was associated with Chadwick in statistical work on public health, but shortly afterwards, his own failing health prevented him from teaching. The university authorities requested Allan Burns to conduct the class, but he refused, and the course was given by Pagan, by this time professor of midwifery at Glasgow. Cowan returned to his duties for a short period in 1841, but died in October of that year, aged 45.

The government, in creating a regius chair at Glasgow, hoped to further university reform while serving political interests. Its commitment went no further, for the regius chair had no salary, and the professor was expected to make his living from student fees, estimated at between £200 and £300 a year, and private practice.[39] Regius professors in Scotland did not expect much endowment—between £50 and £100 was normal, but this chair was to be entirely self-supporting in its early years. A small allowance was made from university funds to provide the professor with an assistant, shared with the professor of materia medica. In this unpromising way, the study of forensic medicine in Glasgow began.

Harry Rainy's appointment as second regius professor in 1841 ushered in a period of relative obscurity for forensic medicine in the University of Glasgow, lasting for 57 years until the retirement of his successor, Pierce Adolphus Simpson. Neither Rainy nor Simpson was actively involved in medico-legal autopsies, or made many appearances in court. Their main contribution was through the teaching of forensic medicine, where they both seem to have been competent, if not distinguished. Edinburgh carried the palm in Scottish forensic medicine until the 1890s, for amongst Sir Robert Christison's successors were men of high standing: two of them, Douglas Maclagan and Henry Littlejohn, received knighthoods.

Several notorious murders took place in Glasgow during this time,[40] including two sensational cases of poisoning. In 1857, Madeleine Smith, an attractive young woman from the higher circles of Glasgow society, was tried for poisoning her lover with arsenic. She was released (though very likely guilty), on a verdict of not proven.[41] In 1865, Edward Pritchard, a disreputable medical man, was tried and hanged for poisoning his wife and mother-in-law with antimony. From these, and other celebrated trials, the Glasgow professors were absent: their colleagues in chemistry or surgery were preferred as local witnesses, but, embarrassingly, if the Crown required expert advice, it looked eastwards. Christison was called in evidence against Madeleine Smith, and although it was proved conclusively that the victim's death was due to arsenical poisoning, the prosecution was not able to prove murder rather than suicide. Maclagen appeared for the defence to offer some credibility to Miss Smith's claim that she had bought arsenic as a beauty aid, to use when washing her face. In the Pritchard case, Maclagan and Littlejohn were called by the Crown. Even a Glasgow historian must reluctantly admit that if the prosecution needed a weighty medical witness in these years, it usually went to Edinburgh to find one.

Edinburgh, like Glasgow, appointed its regius professors by patronage, and its early fame in forensic medicine was partly a matter of luck. Christison, with powerful Tory patrons, succeeded to the chair in his early twenties, without having given any proof of his ability in the subject apart from a youthful fondness for chemistry: his great talent became apparent only after his appointment. He made the chair of forensic medicine so useful to the law courts that all the later appointments in Edinburgh were experienced medical witnesses, most of them working as police surgeons in addition to their university duties. Glasgow was less lucky: political influence did not result in a distinguished appointment.

Harry Rainy was 48 years old when he was appointed to the Glasgow chair in 1841. A son of the manse, he was an able man of wide experience, but his suitability for the post was not obvious. He had taken his degree at Glasgow and became a Fellow of the Royal College of Physicians and Surgeons in 1815. In the same year he went to Paris, where he witnessed the events of the 'hundred days' of Napoleon's return. Rainy worked in the Paris hospitals and studied eye surgery, which he intended to make his career. When he returned to Glasgow, he acquired a large general practice, but his interest in opthalmology remained, and he helped his friend William McKenzie to found the Glasgow Eye Infirmary in 1824. Rainy's head appeared in a medallion on the south front of the infirmary in Berkley Street.

Rainy's first entrance to the university came when he was appointed as a substitute lecturer in the theory of physic for Charles Badham, the professor of medicine. From 1832 to 1839 Rainy taught Badham's classes, for the ultra-conservative Badham, an outstanding valetudinarian, insisted on living in the south of France for the sake of his health. Badham continued to draw his university salary of some £300 per year, and took a quarter of the students' fees, about £150: Rainy took the remaining three-quarters. Rainy's classes were well regarded, and he should have been an obvious candidate for the new regius chair in theory of physic in 1839, but was not to the Whig government's liking. James Oswald, the MP who acted as a broker in these matters, wrote to the Lord Advocate:

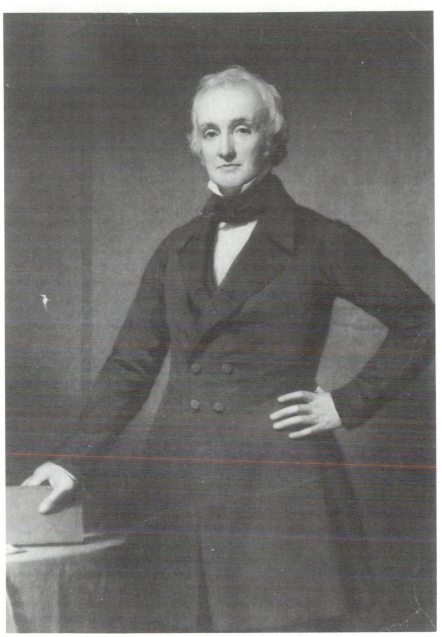

3   Harry Rainy, second Regius Professor (GUA)

> There can no fault be found with Dr. Rennie [sic] as a lecturer, but he is about
> as rabid and intolerant and active a Tory as is in this great City—He is also a
> violent Church Tory and an admirer of Dr. Chalmers, and the most decided enemy
> in all particulars to Her Majesty's present Ministers.[42]

When the new chair was given to Buchanan, Rainy took over the other part
of Badham's duties, teaching the practice of physic, until Badham retired
in 1840. Badham's chair then went to another Whig candidate, William
Thomson, son of the professor of pathology at Edinburgh, who had influence
with the Lord Advocate. Rainy was deliberately excluded from the chair, in
spite of strong support within the University.

The Whig government fell in August 1841 and Sir Robert Peel became
Prime Minister: had Badham clung to his office for only a few extra months,
Rainy would almost certainly have replaced him as professor of medicine.
Instead, it was the vacant chair of forensic medicine, now in the gift of the
Tory party, which was Rainy's consolation prize. As soon as Cowan died,
the Senate approached the government on Rainy's behalf, and the new
appointment was announced within the month.[43]

Rainy's appointment provoked some harsh remarks, not only in the local
press, but in the *Lancet*, which considered the merits of Rainy's rivals for the
chair.[44] Several other candidates with experience of chemistry or forensic
medicine had arguably better claims to expertise in the subject than Rainy.[45]
Such discussions, however, were inevitably coloured by political feelings,
and at that time, all-round competence was often favoured above specialist
knowledge in academic life.

Yet Rainy did not become a practical forensic expert, mainly because of his
difficult temperament. His handsome, erect figure could have made him a
powerful presence in the witness box, but he was not an approachable man,
and was described as impassive and cold by one of his pupils. Another
observed that,

> he was not only cross-looking, but easily made cross. This was an unfortunate
> trait in a Professor of Medical Jurisprudence, whose opinion would naturally
> have been often sought in a court of law; but counsel quickly discovered they
> could make nothing of him in the witness box, and so very soon gave him up
> completely.[46]

Rainy's large general practice, rather than court fees, supplemented his university income.

Rainy's deficiencies as a medical witness did not prevent him from teaching
medical jurisprudence competently. His reputation in the university had been
built on his teaching ability, and once appointed to the chair, he taught
forensic medicine confidently, without notes, and was active in university
administration. His lecture schedule in 1862 shows the dual function of
forensic medicine in the university. Medical students were to be instructed
on the legal responsibilities of their profession, and given basic training on
how to determine the cause of death. Law students should learn the value,

and the limitations, of medical evidence in court. Rainy's course showed none of Cowan's interest in the sanitary aspects of medical police, but concentrated entirely on forensic medicine. Its outline was as follows:

1. Death-bed illness—testamentary ability—Scotch law of deathbed in relation to heritable property—legal definition of deathbed—caution when death is within 60 days disposal of property. 2. Signs of death. 3. Time elapsed since death. 4. Personal identity. 5. Natural or criminal. 6-8. Lightning, cold, starvation. 9. Burning. 10. Poisoning. 11. Respiration. 12. External signs of violence in the living and dead. 13. Sexual functions—Rape—Impotence—Infection. 14. Bodily soundness for Jury duty—Army—Navy. 15. Insanity. 16. Conclusions—duties of medical men in relation to judicial proceedings—duties of legal practitioners in relation to medical evidence whether for prosecution or defence.[47]

Rainy's lectures show the wide-ranging concerns of forensic medicine at this time, not only with crime but with property matters. Criminal detection was only a part of the medical man's legal duties: questions of sanity and deathbed disposals also affected the ownership of property.[48] The old Scottish law of 'deathbed', given some attention in the lectures, permitted legal disputes over wills if the deceased had made the will less than 60 days before death. Unless his heirs could prove that he was sound in mind and body, and not suffering from his last illness at the time of the will, it could be challenged by other claimants. Medical evidence was therefore of much importance in court. This law, not revoked until 1874, was not likely to affect many people, but since it gave the medical profession a particular legal responsibility, nineteenth-century lecture courses always discussed it.

Like most nineteenth-century textbooks, Rainy's lectures were biased towards toxicology, and by 1868 his lecture schedule included fewer legal matters.[49] At the time Rainy taught, any general practitioner could be summoned to perform a post-mortem and carry out basic tests for poisoning. In larger cities like Glasgow and Edinburgh, the fiscal would usually call an experienced police surgeon for post-mortems and a reputable chemist for toxicological analysis. Many a Scottish doctor, however, would be working in smaller communities where the general practitioner was the only available expert: others went to England, where the coroners' courts often summoned the nearest available doctor. Preparation for legal responsibilities had to be part of a medical student's training.

The strong emphasis on toxicology requires a brief comment. Poisons, including narcotics, were readily avilable from apothecaries, and the medical profession itself dispensed many toxic preparations. The use of poisons was virtually uncontrolled in household cleaning fluids, paint, artists' materials, vermin killers, and so forth, as well as being a regular hazard of many trades. Homicidal poisonings were in fact very rare, suicides by poison less so. Poisoning was most likely to be caused by domestic accidents or industrial exposure to toxic material; but, as an instrument of murder, the secret and premeditated use of poison had a powerful hold on the public imagination.

Rainy followed the usual nineteenth-century pattern in making it the central feature of his teaching.

At that time, there were few reliable tests for detecting poison in a body, and the best needed very skillful handling. The most effective chemical tests were for metallic poisons such as arsenic or antimony, which, not being broken down in the body or liable to decay, might be detected in cadavers years after death. Vegetable poisons like opium or strychnine were rapidly destroyed, and much harder to detect. Rainy and other teachers of the time used traditional forms of detection as corroborative evidence, including the characteristic odours given off by poisons during boiling. Analysts also had to be prepared to taste the boiled-down extracts of bodily organs in the search for the bitterness of strychnine or opium.[50] Well into the twentieth century, the taste test for strychnine was still recommended—'with great caution'.[51]

The Marsh test for arsenic required that the suspected substance be mixed with dilute sulphuric acid and zinc to produce a gas of arseniuretted hydrogen. The test was notoriously liable to mislead if the analyst used commercial materials which were themselves contaminated by arsenic, since arsenic was often naturally present in the ores which contained sulphur, copper and zinc. The Reinsch process offered a further preliminary test, in which the suspect fluid was boiled with hydrochloric acid and copper foil, after which the arsenic tarnished the copper with a grey film. Since the analyst could not trust any one test, he was encouraged to carry out as many as possible, both chemical and microscopic, to see if they all agreed—a most laborious business. Nine-teenth-century works on toxicology became increasingly complicated, and the good analyst was known by the complexity of his tests and the numbers of checks he carried out.

Rainy was interested in chemistry, and before his appointment had written some short essays on the specific gravity of hydrogen. As professor, he undertook practical research on Reinsch's process. It was known that the process, though apparently able to detect minute quantities of arsenic, would some-times fail to detect much larger quantities. Rainy's experiments seemed to show that if too large an area of copper was used, small quantities of arsenic would not be able to tarnish it; but, particularly, if the arsenic had been in solution for some time, it formed an acid which was resistant to the Reinsch test. These were practical conclusions, but Rainy's suggestion for enhancing the test's reliability by adding an animal substance such as milk, was not corroborated.[52]

Rainy made a more important contribution to a subject which is still an uncertain part of forensic medicine: the cooling time of dead bodies. In theory, since a dead body cools to the temperature of its environment, a body which retains some animal heat should give a clue to the time of death—a crucial issue in many murder cases. Rainy and his friend Joseph Coats, then lecturer in pathology, carried out observations on dying patients in the Royal Infirmary, trying to find a standard time of cooling in bodies which were in 'still air of uniform temperature'. When a patient died, the temperature in the rectum was taken at hourly intervals until the body reached the same temperature as the ambient air. Newton's Law of Cooling stated that the rate of heat loss from a solid object was directly proportional to the difference in temperature between the object and its environment: that is, if a body lost one-twentieth of its heat between 11 a.m. and noon, it would then lose one-twentieth of its noon temperature by 1 p.m., and so on. By measuring the cooling time once the body was discovered, and then calculating backwards, the time of death could be known. Rainy's measurements on the bodies of 46 patients who had died of a variety of diseases, from phthisis to cancer, showed that the measurements were not so simple. During the nineteenth century, it became known that the bodies of people dying from cholera actually showed a rise in temperature at the time of death: this proved true of certain other diseases, and also of death from asphyxiation. This happened to one of the bodies Rainy observed. In 23 bodies, the rate of cooling per hour increased, being faster during the last five hours than during the first four. In 11 others it was faster at the beginning than the end, though Rainy was not able to explain this, and put it down to heat generated by the beginning of decomposition. Rainy's own mathematical equation, expressed in logarithms, calculated a relationship between the observed cooling time and temperature at death, which allowed the time of death to be deduced.[53] To spare the embarrassment of unscientific practitioners, Rainy added charitably:

> Persons unacquainted with logarithms may make the necessary observations when the body is found, and the proper inference may be deduced by competent parties afterwards.[54]

Since his observations had shown that the body did not cool at a a steady rate, Rainy assumed that the final calculation might underestimate the amount of time since death, because the rate of cooling was normally slower soon after death. He wrote,

> though we cannot calculate exactly the period which has elapsed since death, we can almost always determine a maximum and a minimum of time within which that period will be included, sufficiently close for all practical purposes, in those cases in which the body is found with a temperature in the rectum distinctly above that of the surrounding medium.[55]

Rainy's calculations had a fairly wide margin of error, nor did they take account of complicating factors such as the irregular shape of the human body, which leads to uneven distribution of heat after death, nor of variables like the amount of fat, or clothing. Bodies discovered outdoors would probably be subject to fluctuations in external temperature, unlike the patients in the Royal Infirmary. A precise measurement of time of death based on body temperature has eluded forensic medicine, which must be content with a margin of error of about four hours,[56] but Rainy's researches helped to clarify the problem, and, expressed graphically as 'Rainy's curve', they achieved a wide currency as a 'rule of thumb' measure. Their combination of scientific observation and cautious guesswork is characteristic of modern forensic medicine.

Rainy remained professor until 1872, teaching his students the value of common sense in forensic medicine. Under his tenure, his chair was usually referred to as 'forensic medicine' rather than 'medical jurisprudence', signalling his interest in medical rather than legal subjects. During his time the University moved to its new site on Gilmorehill, away from the crowded city to the select residences of the West End. Rainy died in 1876, leaving a comfortable estate worth £29,438.[57] He left £1,500 in his will to set up bursaries for the benefit of students. His son, the Rev.Robert Rainy, became a prominent figure in the controversies of the Scottish church.

Under Rainy's successor, Pierce Adolphus Simpson, the university's reputation in forensic medicine was not enhanced, though on paper Simpson's qualifications were superior to Rainy's. Born in Ireland in 1837, the youngest son of a landowner in County Leitrim, Simpson was a vigorous man in his mid thirties when appointed to the chair. He had been educated at Rugby and taken the mathematics tripos at Cambridge before turning to medicine. In 1861 he took his MD at Edinburgh, studying under William Tennant Gairdner (soon to become Glasgow's first MOH), and Henry Littlejohn. He then came to Glasgow, where he built up a private practice and took several appointments which were bound to further his career: resident physician at the Royal Infirmary, assistant surgeon at the prison, physician to the Glasgow dispensary for diseases of the chest, and editor of the *Glasgow Medical Journal*. In 1866 he became a Fellow of the Glasgow Faculty of Physicians and Surgeons, and later an examiner in medical jurisprudence for the Faculty's diploma. He became lecturer in medical jurisprudence at the Andersonian medical school in 1866, and two years later was promoted to the Andersonian's chair in that subject. He replaced John Black Cowan, Robert Cowan's son, who in the usual Glasgow game of musical chairs, had been appointed professor of *materia medica* at the University of Glasgow.

Simpson's mathematical mind and his work in medical jurisprudence gave him the opportunity to work for life insurance companies, and he became medical referee for the Scottish Provincial and Scottish Commercial Assurance Association. This was a lucrative business, with a fee of a guinea or more for a short examination of each prospective policy holder. So well regarded was this kind of work amongst the profession that lectures in medical jurisprudence often included advice to students on how to conduct life insurance examinations.[58] Simpson was also a factory certifying surgeon, examining cases of industrial injury, and in later life he became consulting physician for the British Home for Incurables (Scotland).[59] His private practice in the West End flourished, and his financial success was further assured when he married a wealthy wife, Frances Adelaide Leisler.

When Simpson was appointed to the chair of forensic medicine at Glasgow University, his testimonials were even more inflated than most documents of their type, and showed a promising young man who had already secured his position in Glasgow society.[60] During Rainy's time, the political heat had gone out of university appointments, and although Simpson was a Conservative, he was appointed by Gladstone's Liberal government. The real influence over appointments had passed to the Senate and the new Court of the reformed

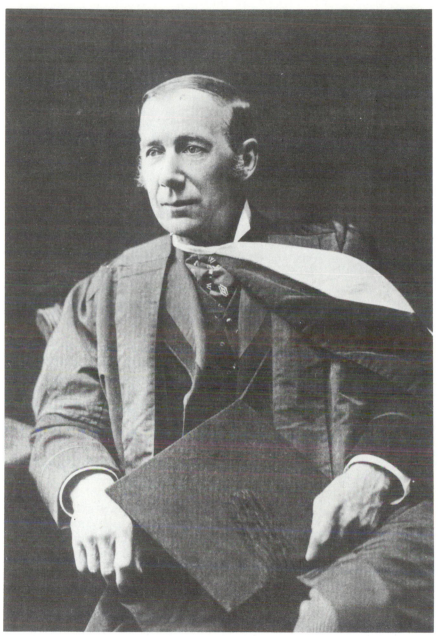

4   Pierce Adolphus Simpson, third Regius Professor (GUA)

university. The candidates for the chair now needed to offer more than political credentials.

Henry Littlejohn, who supported Simpson's application, commented that a professor of forensic medicine would probably become a Crown witness, but there is no evidence that Simpson ever attempted this. Post-mortem work and court appearances were time-consuming, and Simpson had little need of the fees, preferring to cultivate his private practice and other well-paid interests. Known disrespectfully to his students as 'Paddy', Simpson was a genial man, a *bon viveur*, and a member of several gentlemen's clubs. He was also a refined and liberal supporter of the arts, and, it seems, generally too busy for serious work in forensic medicine. His only publications appear to be an article on 'old age' in the *Transactions of the Insurance and Actuarial Society of Glasgow*, and two addresses to students.

Four student notebooks of Simpson's lectures survive to show how forensic medicine was taught in the later nineteenth century.[61] Simpson's course consisted of 46 lectures, and he taught every day during the summer term. Forensic medicine became a part of the law curriculum in 1864, and Simpson taught law and medical students separately. The course for law students was offered in alternate years, and was given in the Philosophical Society's rooms at 207 Bath Street. Nineteenth-century students had relatively few textbooks (Simpson's classes used A.S. Taylor's standard text on medical jurisprudence),[62] and lectures were delivered slowly, enabling the class to take very full notes. These would also be the basis of the weekly 'examination', and at the end of the course, the students would elect the winner of the class prize. The notes were written out very formally in bound notebooks, and students often took the trouble to make a fair copy, embellished by different coloured inks, elaborate capital letters and other fanciful decorations.[63] There is little obvious difference, apart from more attention to the identification of bloodstains, between the structure or content of Simpson's course at different dates in his career. This may indicate a certain inertia on the lecturer's part, although few academics would care to be judged on the quality of their students' lecture notes.

Simpson's course followed Taylor's textbook, and its outline in 1879 consisted of: the definition of death; time since death; means of identifying a body; death from starvation, cold, sunstroke, burns, etc; deaths from asphyxia; wounds; poisons; rape; legitimacy (i) viability (ii) impotence; infanticide (i) delivery (ii) concealment of pregnancy; survivorship; insanity; medical examinations for life insurance; legal duties of medical men.[64] In fact, Simpson devoted much of the course to the appearance of the body after death, probable cause of death, and toxicology. On the question of rape and virginity, the Professor was apparently philosophical, as his student noted in 1883:

> Virginity. What is it? Is it a moral virtue or is it something of a physical kind, and if it is of a physical kind, what are the signs?[65]

Like other teachers on this subject, Simpson was anxious to point out to his students that there were no infallible answers.

In the last years of his tenure, Simpson suffered from ill-health, and lectures were given by Donald Munro, his assistant for 23 years. In 1897 the Senate appointed Hugh Galt, later professor of medical jurisprudence at St. Mungo's, to undertake Simpson's work, and Simpson himself was at last persuaded to retire in 1898. He died in 1900, with an estate valued at £42,060—a very comfortable fortune. He had not earned it from his university work. Although his chair still carried no salary when he accepted it, university reform in the later nineteenth century commuted his student fees into a fixed salary of around £600.[66] As Simpson had not increased this with earnings from court work, it was his private practice, family money and other appointments which made him a comparatively wealthy man. Although he was a popular figure in Glasgow, his early promise in forensic medicine had not been fulfilled, and he appears a *dilettante* in comparison with his contemporaries in Edinburgh. In 1898 all this changed. John Glaister was appointed to the regius chair, and forensic medicine became a very serious business.

CHAPTER TWO

John Glaister I: The Professor

Oh I am the marvel of Medical Ju.
A fact which I've tried to impress upon you,
I never get flurried, whatever I do,
For I'm the great Professor John Glaister
Just bear that in mind and you're sure to get through.[1]

The name of John Glaister the elder (1856-1932) is familiar to every generation of medical students in the University of Glasgow through convivial
recitations of the *Ballad of John Glaister*, which is often attributed to Osborne
Mavor (James Bridie) and some of his fellow students. Variants of this lengthy
piece have spread to many lands: the appeal of its antique obscenities is
unfailing. For some time, a copy hung on a common-room wall in Harvard
medical school, leading some students to suppose that Glaister was a fictional
character like Sherlock Holmes.[2] Despite its scabrous expression, the *Ballad*
gives a fair indication of the catholic interests of a professor of forensic
medicine in the heroic age of the subject. It refers to sudden death, sexual
perversions, elementary psychology, problematic consummation of marriage,
abortion, rape, toxicology, fingerprints, drunkenness, the construction of
privies and the disposal of effluent. John Glaister considered himself expert in
all these fields.

The ballad reflects the contents of Glaister's *Textbook of Medical Jurisprudence, Toxicology and Public Health*, published in 1902. Glaister was the last
professor in the department to combine the teaching of forensic medicine and
public health, according to the old Scottish convention of medical police. He
was also the first professor to act as medico-legal examiner for the Crown,
and it was his forensic work which established his international reputation.
Yet the development of forensic medicine in Scotland can only be understood
in relation to its connection with public health, and it was expertise in public
health which brought Glaister the chair. An account of his career should
properly begin with this part of his work.

Now please understand I'm a self-made M.D.
I'm a D.P.H. Cantab. and F.R.S.E.

Glaister was born in Lanark in 1856, the eldest of the four children of Joseph Glaister and Marion Hamilton Weir. His parents were small property holders, with a business as grocers and wine and spirit merchants on the ground floor of one of the tenements they owned. Glaister reputedly finished his education at Lanark Grammar School a year early and spent the next year as a pupil teacher.[3] This post allowed him access to a locked bookcase, a source of much furtive interest to the boys. It contained papers and anatomical drawings on midwifery by William Smellie, the eighteenth-century pioneer of obstetrics: Smellie, also a former pupil, had left his papers to the school. This discovery had a strong influence on Glaister, then and later: more than twenty years afterwards, he was to write Smellie's biography.[4]

The years following his schooldays were difficult. In 1871, aged 15, he was apprenticed to the law. His parents and a younger brother died shortly afterwards, and since their father had died intestate while the children were still minors, they were placed under the care of their uncle, Thomas Glaister. He bought the family property and business, and this probably provided funds for their upbringing. John Glaister then decided to leave his law apprenticeship and enter the University of Glasgow to study medicine, which may have attracted him the more because of the deaths of his parents, as well as his early interest in Smellie's papers.[5]

Glaister was an exceptionally gifted student who carried off many prizes and completed his studies in less than four years, but he was refused permission to sit the professional M.B. examinations because he was still some months under the regulation age of 21. Undeterred, he obtained diplomas from the two Edinburgh Royal Colleges in 1877 and worked as assistant to a practitioner in Carluke for six months before setting up for himself in Townhead. Glaister finally took his medical degree in Glasgow in 1879.[6]

In those days, Deans of medicine did not hesitate to offer their students advice on intimate matters, and one piece of counsel given at an opening address to the medical students around this time was that doctors should not marry until they were established in their careers. Heedless of such advice, Glaister married Mary Scott Clarke in 1878, and they set up house in Grafton Place, with a surgery in St Mungo Street, Townhead. With the arrival in 1879 of Isabella, the first of their six children, Glaister had even more incentive to establish himself professionally. Townhead in the 1880s was a bustling, thriving district, and Glaister soon worked up a good family practice. However, as he said, he was 'early bent towards medical teaching.'[7]

Glaister was a 'self-made' man in that he had no powerful family patrons, nor had he the advantages enjoyed by some of the outstanding figures in Scottish forensic medicine. Robert Christison, for example, was the son of a professor, had travelled widely in Europe, studied toxicology in Paris, and read both French and German. Glaister's education was more provincial, but his circle of friends included many enterprising young Glasgow doctors, amongst whom he made valuable friendships. One influential friend was William Macewen, just beginning his rise to surgical fame. At that time, Macewen was a general practitioner in Glaister's district and a police surgeon in the Central division. He and Glaister conferred with one another on difficult cases. Macewen lectured on medical jurisprudence in the Glasgow Royal Infirmary Medical School (soon to become St Mungo's College), and Glaister assisted him. Glaister may well have studied pathology and medical jurisprudence under Macewen,[8] and he also taught toxicology under Macewen's direction. When Macewen took a lectureship in surgery at the Royal Infirmary, Glaister succeeded him as lecturer in medical jurisprudence in May 1881.

In the mid 1880s Glaister introduced lectures on public health into his medical jurisprudence course at the Royal Infirmary. Public health was then highly topical. Many English and Scottish medical corporations and universities were instituting postgraduate degrees and diplomas following the 1875 Public Health Act, which made it compulsory for local authorities south of the border to appoint Medical Officers of Health. All three Scottish medical licensing corporations awarded Diplomas in Public Health (DPH) by 1889. Although public health had been taught with medical jurisprudence in the extra-mural schools at Glasgow and Edinburgh, it was not examined separately until 1875, with Littlejohn at the Edinburgh extra-mural school, followed by Christie at the Andersonian in 1879: Aberdeen University also offered a course of practical hygiene lectures under Matthew Hay. In each case public health was taught in combination with forensic medicine.[9]

Scottish medical education was responding to the new demand for doctors qualified in public health. From 1886 the General Medical Council also recognised the DPH,[10] and in 1888 the Local Government Act made it a compulsory qualification for Medical Officers of Health in large local authorities. From 1889 the same provisions applied to Scotland. Scottish doctors were a migratory breed, and medical students saw the DPH as a qualification likely to improve their prospects for a career in public service in many parts of the world.

The department of forensic medicine in Glasgow in the late nineteenth century seemed to be an oddity. Despite his chair's origins in concern over public health, Harry Rainy's syllabus never included the study of hygiene. W T Gairdner may have included some medical police subjects in his own lectures as professor of medicine, and, as MOH for the city from 1863 to 1872, he was more qualified to do so than Rainy. From 1872 he lectured on fevers and contagion, and organised practical visits to the municipal fever hospitals.[11]

Simpson, who had no great reputation in forensic medicine, managed to achieve notoriety in public health.[12] In 1889 he involved the university in a scandal which aroused the wrath of the General Medical Council and brought the university's DPH into disrepute. Simpson's chief critic in the affair was Glaister, by then Professor of Medical Jurisprudence and Public Health at St Mungo's. Glaister's shadow thus fell on the department almost a decade before he became its fourth regius professor.

Simpson, whose lectures were patterned on A S Taylor's textbook, concentrated on forensic medicine and was not interested in public health. He seems to have been aroused by events at Edinburgh, where, in addition to the established undergraduate teaching of medical police with forensic medicine, two postgraduate degrees in public health were instituted in 1875.[13]

Simpson decided to match Edinburgh's entrepreneurial action by setting up his own version of the DPH, but from 1876 to 1888 only four candidates took the examination.[14]

Meanwhile the GMC was trying to impose some uniformity on the plethora of public health qualifications offered in Britain. It set certain standards, including laboratory instruction with a stipulated amount of microscopy. To meet these requirements, Glaister was appointed in 1887 as special lecturer in public health at the Royal Infirmary, with a laboratory which he equipped at his own expense. He also built many of the practical models himself. This was the only public health laboratory in Glasgow to teach at a sufficiently high standard for the Cambridge DPH (considered the most prestigious), and for the three Scottish licensing bodies.[15]

The GMC prodded Glasgow University Senate to conform to acceptable standards for the DPH, and Simpson was asked to set up a more regular course, but he was hampered because he had no laboratory. The Senate, against the advice of the GMC, also relaxed the regulations so that students could take the DPH examination with their final professional examinations, instead of undertaking postgraduate study. The first examination of this kind was in 1889, just as the Local Government Act was creating a larger number of appointments for holders of the DPH. Fifty-five candidates presented themselves for the examination, and all passed.

At this point Glaister protested to the GMC about the low standard of the university examination, comparing it unfavourably with examination papers from other institutions. The two Glasgow papers were innocent of questions on epidemiology, communicable diseases, sanitary law, vital statistics, or dietetics. There was no practical examination on the analysis of air, water, or food, nor any test of microscopy in public health subjects, nor any reports on external visits. These were normal requirements for DPH candidates elsewhere, and it is indeed hard to see how an efficient medical officer of health could have managed without them.[16]

The university defended its position vigorously but unsuccessfully. The GMC censured it and refused to place any future DPHs from Glasgow on the Medical Register until the examinations were reformed. The university therefore invited the original candidates to sit an amended examination. Five accepted, and four passed.[17] Despite the university's hostility, Glaister insisted on raising the awkward question of the graduates with dubious DPHs awarded by Glasgow in 1889 and already placed on the Medical Register. About 20 doctors were involved, some of whom were practising overseas. Glaister's tenacity forced an extraordinary meeting of the university's General Council.[18] He wanted the DPHs rescinded by Act of Parliament, a costly, lengthy and embarrassing process, but the candidates had not been guilty of any professional misconduct, and could not be removed from the Register. In the end, the GMC and the university were unwilling 'to have this old scandal again thrashed out',[19] and the subject was quietly dropped. The best that can be said of Simpson's part in the affair is that approaching ill-health may have clouded his judgement.

In the 1890s, Glaister wrote a book and several articles on public health, which seemed his major interest.[20] When Simpson retired in January 1898, Glaister applied for the chair, his testimonials stressing his expertise in teaching public health. The university apparently bore no grudges, and appointed him: able men with special qualifications in both public health and forensic medicine were hard to find.

Once again the chair's passing from one regius professor to the next focused attention on its teaching responsibilities. The University Court wished to separate forensic medicine from public health completely, pointing out to the Secretary for Scotland that in public health great progress had been made and much legislation passed since the appointment of the last professor. In 1897 Edinburgh had already separated the two subjects and created a new chair of public health:[21] Simpson's retiral offered an opportunity for Glasgow to do the same. The argument which then took place within the government of the university reveals some of the perennial difficulties in maintaining forensic medicine as a university discipline.

By the end of the century, the university saw public health as a subject more relevant than forensic medicine to a medical career. The Court wanted two separate chairs, but had no finance for a chair in public health. As an insurance against the creation of a chair in public health, the Court suggested that a clause be inserted into the commission of the new professor to exclude him from teaching public health if a separate chair ever came into being.[22] The Senate wished to go even further, and argued that if a new chair of public health were founded, no chair in forensic medicine would be necessary, and the post could be reduced to a lectureship. The medical faculty, knowing that there were no funds for a new chair, recommended instead that the next regius professor should continue to teach both subjects, but wanted the lectures on public health to be expanded to fill half the course of fifty lectures. It also argued for a properly equipped laboratory, and requested that the Crown take special notice of the public health qualifications of candidates for the new appointment.[23]

Not for the first or last time, the status of forensic medicine within the university was in danger. In the 1890s this may not have seemed unreasonable, since the holders of the chair had not established any great reputation for their subject, whereas public health had strong claims to consideration. Nevertheless, the implication that forensic medicine was a minority interest, or a less important part of the medical curriculum, would have reduced it to the inferior position which it usually occupied in English medical schools.

Glaister was appointed Professor of Forensic Medicine and Public Health on a consensus of these views. His commission did contain the clause on public health teaching, but he was empowered to teach medical jurisprudence to law students, and both medical jurisprudence and public health to medical students. Forensic medicine remained a compulsory part of the medical curriculum. He brought as a dowry the contents of the public health laboratory from St Mungo's, and the university also allowed him around £200 for extra equipment in the separate classes for the newly arrived female students at Queen Margaret College.[24]

Before 1898 the medico-legal laboratory had received little attention, but

Glaister began immediately to keep two separate laboratories for forensic medicine and public health: he ordered green window blinds in order to show limelight slides to his forensic medicine class, and hired a boy to attend to the public health laboratory at 7s.6d. per week. From these small beginnings the technical and laboratory staff developed. In 1903, Glaister began teaching the first B.Sc. and D.Sc. degrees in public health at Glasgow. In 1907 he also taught the men and women students together, arguing that it was advantageous to the women, though he was no doubt happy to give up travelling to the women's college for separate classes. The classes in forensic medicine, considered particularly indelicate for a female audience, were regarded by both staff and male students as a test of feminine nerves.

The public health syllabus took up most space in the department's entry in the university calendar from 1898 to 1923. Courses, laboratory work, fieldwork and recommended textbooks proliferated, while the entry for forensic medicine seemed comparatively static. More staff were needed to cope with the increasing responsibilities, and in the early years of the twentieth century the nucleus of a modern department appeared. In 1908 George A Brown was appointed as an assistant, joined in 1909 by Andrew Allison. Brown left in 1912, and was replaced by Ernest Watt. These assistants all had the DPH qualification, but Allison also specialised in forensic medicine, and was promoted to senior assistant in 1912. He remained in the department until 1921, when he became Lecturer (later Professor) in Forensic Medicine and Public Health at St Mungo's. Until the 1920s the department consisted of Glaister and two assistants; apart from his undergraduate classes in forensic medicine, Glaister taught all postgraduate classes in public health, and in 1917-18 he taught all the courses in both subjects while his assistants were away on war service.

After 1918, returning servicemen flooded into the medical schools, creating havoc with the limited manpower and teaching space. Post-war changes in medical education meant that medical jurisprudence and public health had to be taught separately. The two separate courses, and many more students, quadrupled the department's teaching. Laboratory instruction went on continuously from 9 a.m. to 5 p.m. during both terms. In addition, Glaister taught forensic medicine to law students and the examining burden for both faculties was heavy. In September 1922 Glaister read 590 examination papers and gave 295 oral examinations: the orals alone took ten days, with candidates appearing from 9 a.m. until after 6 p.m.[25]

The increasing work came at the zenith of Glaister's career as a medical witness, and at a time when forensic medicine was undergoing many technical changes. He therefore decided to give up teaching public health. In 1922 he explained his decision in a letter to the Court:

> The time has arrived when in this university the subjects should be separated, and that the department of public health should come under the charge of one who should devote himself exclusively to that subject, leaving me some more time to devote myself to forensic medicine with which my name is particularly associated in this and in other countries.[26]

Glaister made no secret of the fact that he was responsible for obtaining the Henry Mechan chair of public health in 1923.[27] Mechan, an old acquaintance of Glaister's, and a fellow stalwart of the Conservative party, owned a local engineering firm. In the course of a conversation, Glaister told him of the difficulty of balancing his departmental commitments with his court work. Mechan's subsequent offer of £25,000 to endow a chair ended the traditional relationship between public health and forensic medicine in the university. The department of forensic medicine had to give up some of its space to the new department, and the two professors engaged in regular territorial disputes with the ferocious politeness of Samurai warriors.[28] The relationship between the two subjects had established forensic medicine as an integral part of Scottish medical education, and won for it a more secure place than in any English university. Once separated from public health, forensic medicine would have to stand alone and maintain its claims as a necessary part of the university structure. By 1923, Glaister was convinced that his own reputation as a medical witness, together with the modern scientific laboratory which he had established, would safeguard the future of his subject.

> With my wonted cheroot to the windward I stand
> And I wade through the weevils with dexterous hand,
> And by zephyrs of calcium chloride I'm fanned,
> As I pickle each putrid and pultaceous viscus,
> With portions of coffin and neighbouring land.

When Glaister was appointed to the chair in 1898 he was bent on making changes. The physical aspects of the department were scrutinised and found wanting. When the university moved from the Old College in High Street in the centre of Glasgow in 1871 to the Gilbert Scott buildings on the more select Gilmorehill, the department of forensic medicine was housed in the east quadrangle, known as the medical quadrangle. The department had a lecture theatre, a retiring room for the professor, a small storeroom on the entresol floor above, and a large room on the basement floor. There was no proper laboratory, though work may have been carried out in the laboratories of other departments, such as pathology. Glaister considered his department to be 'most inadequately equipped',[29] and set about improving it. With the basement room now containing equipment from St Mungo's public health laboratory, Glaister quickly found himself a place on the university committee for planning laboratory accommodation in the new medical extension between the university and the Western Infirmary.

The new medical buildings were opened by the Prince and Princess of Wales in 1907, amidst decorous academic festivities, and forensic medicine moved into the purpose-built accommodation it was to occupy for the next

40 years. Glaister originally hoped for separate forensic medicine and public health laboratories on two floors, but his first plan was reduced from two full floors to one which gave the department the second and attic floors of the physiology building. It shared an arched entrance and lecture theatre with materia medica, but each had separate laboratories. The attic floor housed the departmental museum and library.

At that time the department was amongst the best equipped in Britain. It was bright, airy and modern. The lecture theatre was in the traditional curved shape; it had a professor's desk and curved demonstration bench with gas and water taps, sinks and electricity sockets. Lectures could be illustrated by lantern slides illuminated by electricity rather than limelight, and the large windows and skylight were darkened with blinds when necessary. The space under the steeply rising seats of the lecture theatre was used for a preparation room, well provided with lockers, cupboards, presses and drawers.

The laboratories were equally well lighted and equipped. The main medico-legal laboratory, termed 'toxicological laboratory', was illuminated by eight double windows, under which ran a continuous bench used for microscopic, spectrosopic and other demonstrations. There were three workbenches with hot and cold water, sinks, steam nozzles, gas-taps and electric sockets. The cold water taps were modified to allow two workers to operate distillation apparatus simultaneously. Specialised washing facilities for the laboratory apparatus were provided, and a room for fumigation had its own internal ventilation hood and exhaust outlet. The laboratory could also be partitioned for use by assistants or students, and had a photographic dark room adjoining. The public health section of the department had a chemical laboratory, a bacteriological laboratory, and a balance room. In short, the new laboratory of 1907 was the result of Glaister's 24 years in forensic medicine and public health. It bore some of the stamp of the nineteenth century, but was essentially a forward-looking twentieth century creation. By 1928, when the Rockefeller Institute investigated the international provision of medico-legal education, the Glasgow laboratory appeared among the most advanced in the world, and it certainly had no competitors in England.[30]

On the attic floor, Glaister created a museum and library which were always open to students. This was a long, impressive room with an arched ceiling, into which were set two rows of curved skylights. Bookshelves lined the walls between the window bays, and were intersected at right angles by cabinets holding such objects as murder weapons, bullets, casts of footprints, and pieces of interestingly fractured skulls. Each bay held a glass-topped case containing photographic illustrations, coloured drawings, or dried medico-legal specimens. There were locked poison cabinets and a revolving frame illustrating typical poisonous plants in their dried form.

By 1928, Glaister could boast that every item in the museum came from his personal collection, gathered over 30 years as medico-legal advisor to the Crown.[31] The medical detectives of the time collected souvenirs in a rather cavalier manner, and were not always scrupulous about asking permission. An Edinburgh student magazine recorded in verse some similar activities of Harvey Littlejohn:

> Two bodies found in a lonely mere,
> Converted into adipocere.
> Harvey, when called in to see 'em,
> Said, 'Just what I need for my museum.'[32]

The department was designed to give the students practical examples, as far as possible. Whether they were general practitioners or consultants, doctors might find themselves called to give expert evidence in court, even though few had first-hand knowledge of forensic medicine, or of court procedure for medical witnesses. Few students would become police surgeons, prison doctors, or work in a department of forensic medicine. It was therefore necessary for them to learn what they could of the subject from museum specimens, lantern slides, and other visual methods. Glaister took students in pairs, selected by student ballot, to assist with post-mortems, and he also arranged for them to visit the courts on days when he was appearing, to see an expert witness in action. His belief in the visual method and instructive example led him to reinforce his teaching by producing a new form of textbook.

> If you butcher your bastards in some lonely nook,
> If you hang up your wife on an opportune hook,
> If you throttle your tailor or sandbag your cook,
> Then I'll track you down with the aid of Bertillon's
> Remarkable scheme, criticised in my book.

Most medical men know Glaister's name through his textbook, which has been in print for some 87 years and through 13 editions. It is not the longest-running British text of its kind, for that honour belongs to A S Taylor's *Principles and Practice of Medical Jurisprudence* (1865), but, like Taylor, it became a standard work in British forensic medicine.

When Glaister came to the department, the university calendar recommended only one textbook in forensic medicine: Guy and Ferrier's *Principles of Forensic Medicine*.[33] There were relatively few textbooks on the subject in English, and most had the same disadvantage: they described relevant cases but had few pictorial illustrations. To fill this gap in presentation Glaister introduced his students to Hofmann's *Atlas of Legal Medicine*.[34] The *Atlas* had lavish photographs and coloured engravings, but no pretensions other than as a handbook of illustrations. There was a demand for a reliable and well-illustrated general textbook.

Glaister's first edition of *Medical Jurisprudence*, published in 1902, still followed the Scottish tradition of combining forensic medicine with public health.[35] The first edition of *Medical Jurisprudence* was highly successful. Its clear format was well supported by photographs, many taken by Glaister himself or under his direction. Glaister was quick to grasp the significance of the rapidly-changing art of photography for his own subject, and adopted

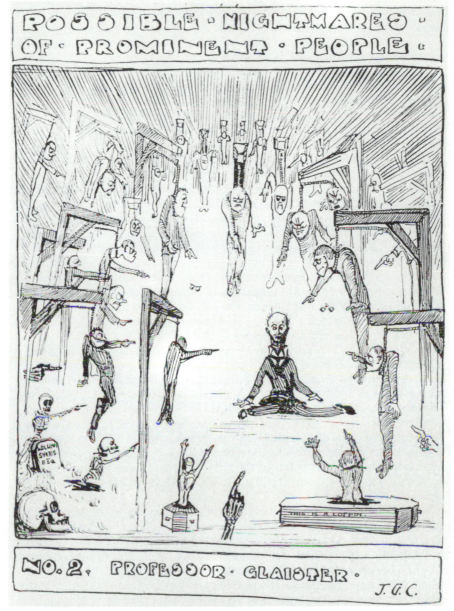

5 A student cartoon of John Glaister with the accusing figures of men he helped to hang (*Glasgow University Magazine*)

new camera techniques enthusiastically. His photographs of the victims of violent crime added to the text a painful realism far removed from the decorous line-drawings of the nineteenth century; but he also used the available techniques of photo-micography to show the features of a single hair which had been forcibly pulled from a scalp, or to reveal an elegant pattern of crystals of arsenious oxide on a tiny piece of wallpaper.

Textbooks in this subject conventionally began with an account of the doctor's legal obligations, but Glaister also paid particular attention to the differences between Scottish and English law. He then considered criminal identification, an area in which he had special interest, having been introduced to it by the Glasgow pioneer of fingerprint techniques, Henry Faulds.[36] Several famous miscarriages of justice had occurred because the courts accepted unreliable evidence based on the elastic memories of policemen and eyewitnesses: Glaister's book described the latest, and most effective techniques of identification. By the end of the nineteenth century, Bertillon's anthropometric system of identifying criminals had been tried by a few police forces in Britain. This included a cumbersome series of twelve measurements of the body, including head, foot, arm and ear, but it was rapidly superseded by identification through fingerprints, a system suggested by Francis Galton and given practical application by Edward R Henry.[37] Glaister's was the first textbook to devote a large section to fingerprint classification, and the reviewers applauded this. Although Glaister believed that doctors must understand all aspects of forensic science, the classification of fingerprints was one of the many skills which would soon belong to the police expert.

In the three succeeding editions of his book (1910, 1915 and 1921), Glaister kept its basic plan, and amended the text to take account of changes in serology, identification of hairs and fibres, ballistics and toxicology. The book thickened as he added yet more examples and photographs from his own experience, and the fourth edition reached 900 pages. Like his visual teaching aids, the descriptions of his cases were intended to give the student graphic illustration of the uses of forensic medicine. Those who studied Glaister's earlier editions differ in their opinion of his tactics. Hard-pressed students with examinations in mind sometimes found the book far too long and detailed for a satisfactory introduction to the subject: others were fascinated by the author's case histories, which still make 'Glaister' compulsive reading for the layman.

Glaister enlivened his lectures with similar anecdotes from his enormous experience of medico-legal affairs. Forensic medicine enthralled many students, and some embarked on their own projects. While he was Glaister's student, E P Cathcart, later famous for his work on nutrition, studied hands for the characteristic occupational markings which could help to identify engineers, hammermen, riveters, violinists, tailors and many others.[38] Those who experienced Glaister's lectures remember his forceful style. Although his subject was compulsory, he did not rely on this to keep the interest of his audience, whereas some of his less fortunate English colleagues, teaching a non-compulsory subject, expected an attentive class only during the annual lecture on rape.

Glaister, unlike his predecessors in the chair, brought to his students the immediacy of his work as chief medico-legal examiner for Glasgow and the county of Lanark. This populous region, in which were found all the social problems of rapid industrialisation, provided him with the raw material for his laboratory and his book, and for the court work which was to establish a durable link between the university and the life of the city.

CHAPTER THREE

John Glaister I: The Complete Medical Detective

Yes, the P.M's the place I exhibit my art,
I carefully carve each particular part,
And the copious notes I make from the start,
Can only be used to refresh my memory,[1]
And in grammar and style are remarkably smart...

If a stairhead encounter is raging apace,
If your Mother-in-law bites chunks off your face,
I can tell from the notes I take on the case,
I can tell from the lesions I find on the body
The time and the tool and the manner and place.

Glaister's first practical experience in forensic medicine came from his work as police surgeon in the St Rollox division of the Glasgow police from 1881. Here he saw the effects on the human body of a wide range of crimes and accidents. An account of the work of a Glasgow police surgeon was given a few years previously by Glaister's colleague, James Dunlop of the Central Division, who reported that, out of 404 cases in three years (nearly one-third of which involved cadavers), around half had serious wounds:

> These wounds varied in position, in size, and in severity. Some of them were large, ragged, and upon the scalp, and were usually produced by falls either down stairs or upon the street; others small and upon the face, inflicted by falls or weapons, such as pokers, sticks, glass bottles, &c. Some were clean and deep cuts in the belly or thighs with knives or stillettos, or on the wrists by the hands being pushed through panes of glass; others were ragged, torn, bruised wounds, inflicted by toothed wheels of machinery, by railway buffers, or cart wheels, etc.[2]

Glaister's experience was similar, and since his district also included the Forth and Clyde canal, he examined many bodies taken from the water; he could therefore distinguish between wounds inflicted during life, and those caused after death by the screws of passing steamers. By 1893 he calculated that he had seen around 300 dead bodies as part of his duties, though he complained that the economical habits of the procurator fiscal prevented his carrying out post-mortems on as many of them as he would have wished.[3]

Glaister had to resign his duties as a police surgeon on moving from

Townhead, but he knew that if he were appointed to the chair he would immediately be offered regular court work in the Lower Ward of the County of Lanark, including Glasgow. Thereafter he preferred to style himself Medico-legal Examiner in Crown cases. This was not a formal appointment, but meant that Glaister expected to be called by the fiscal as a matter of course whenever special expertise was required. In Scotland the fiscals still guard their customary right to call any medical man they please for legal purposes, but in practice there was, and is, a list of doctors with forensic skill who are summoned when necessary. Scarcely a year into his professorship, Glaister became second in the Lanarkshire list, when he was called to work alongside Dunlop, then professor of surgery at the Andersonian. Since two doctors were required to report in all serious cases, both were called into court, though the senior doctor usually took most of the responsibility in the witness box. After two years Glaister succeeded Dunlop as senior examiner, and for the rest of his career he gave medical evidence in all notable criminal trials in the West of Scotland, not only in his own district, but in the neighbouring ones, and in many other courts as well. As his obituary in the *BMJ* noted:

> Professor Glaister's name became a household word, as every newspaper with more or less sensationalism published spicy extracts from his evidence in all the criminal trials for nearly a generation.[4]

On his appointment to the chair, Glaister demonstrated his dedication to forensic medicine by selling his Townhead practice to his brother Joseph. From 1892, Scottish university professors no longer relied on fees from students as a major source of income, but were guaranteed a minimum salary by the university: medical professors expected to supplement this by taking private patients. Glaister, however, earned extra money only from medico-legal work—two guineas for a post-mortem, a guinea or more a day for appearing in court, and about two guineas per session if he spent more than two hours a day on analysis of productions.[5] He also charged for visits to prisons and mental homes to investigate the sanity of those about to stand trial. Like Simpson, he acted as medical referee for life insurance companies: investigating the health of prospective clients at a guinea a time was better paid than conducting a post-mortem. His work supported him very comfortably, and he continued to enjoy an affluent style of life, buying a house in a fashionable part of the West End of Glasgow, and later a small country estate in Dumfriesshire. He was well supplied with servants, kept an excellent table, and indulged his passion for motoring.[6]

In spite of his professional duties, Glaister found time to read papers to learned societies, dabble in history and archaeology, organise university ceremonies and choirs, and be a pillar of the St Rollox Conservative Association. For many years he was an active member of the Glasgow Southern Medical Society, to whom he addressed frequent lectures on public health. It has been well said that the Edwardian years were 'a golden age of comfortable living and high status, when professors were still grandees in local society as well as in their university.'[7]

Glaister proved himself a master of empirical medical detection, based on close observation and careful reasoning. To a public eagerly awaiting each new appearance of Sherlock Holmes, men like Spilsbury, Glaister and the Littlejohns were fascinating. They placed the stamp of scientific respectability on a discipline which had not always won the confidence of either the lawyers or the public. The medical detectives presented the work of scientists to the public in the same way as the performing artist presents the work of the composer. In Glaister's case, his performance also established his university department as an important centre of medico-legal activity. Glaister had a relatively firm base in a university: Spilsbury, with various personal lectureships in London hospitals, had not.[8] Nor did Glaister allow his talent for public performance to eclipse his interest in the teamwork of basic science: as will be seen, he encouraged scientific research in the growing department of the 1920s. He was also at an advantage by having few rivals in Glasgow: the city police had no official laboratory until they set up a fingerprint department in 1931,[9] and other medico-legal inquiries had to be carried out in hospitals or private surgeries. The new laboratory in the university was by far the best equipped to carry out scientific tests, and the police made heavy use of it.

Glaister worked in a well-planned laboratory in the university, but carried out his post-mortems under quite different conditions. No resources had been devoted to civic mortuaries, and Glaister worked in various makeshift rooms, including the top floor of the central police station, and ramshackle out-buildings elsewhere. Each township in Lanarkshire expected the medical expert to come when needed, but gave him minimal assistance. Conditions in outlying districts were particularly bad, with Hamilton notorious for its leaking roof, insanitary facilities and the difficulty in keeping out inquiring members of the public.

A case in the Glasgow circuit court in March 1899, in which Glaister appeared for the defence, shows the kind of expertise which caught the attention of the Crown authorities. A young labourer was accused of murdering his elderly landlady, who appeared to have been struck across the face with a flat, broad weapon, kicked with heavy boots, and had hair pulled from her head. The Crown's medical evidence strongly supported this version of events. Glaister, by using the Crown's own evidence and visiting the scene of the crime, reconstructed a different version:

> The room of the assault was next examined. It had been left exactly as it was found by the police. There was no appearance of any struggle. On the wood facing of the window, which had a comparatively sharp edge, about $2\frac{3}{4}$ feet from the floor we found a slight indentation in the wood, and in its neighbourhood certain marks of blood—viz. running floorwards from the indentation was a tiny stream of blood which had dried, and around the indentation were circular and inverted soda-water-bottle-shaped marks of blood, the latter of which, especially, pointed to the fact that the blood had been forcibly projected against the woodwork from a point close to the woodwork. In addition, on the window facing were irregular, thin smears of blood, in two of which were found hairs which were detached and taken for examination. Close to the wooden facing on which

the blood-spots were found stood a wickerwork arm-chair covered with a light-coloured chintz, on the extremities of which, at a point where the hands of a person seated in a chair would naturally rest on attempting to rise, were bloody finger-marks and smears.[10]

Glaister surmised that the old lady fell against the window frame of a dark upstairs bedroom, injuring her face to such an extent that, dazed, she raised herself by using a chair and a chest of drawers and sank on to her bed, where she lay for a short time: she then got up and tried to go downstairs, but fell down the sharply-angled flight, breaking her ribs: the signs of this progress could also be seen from marks on the stairs. Glaister identified the Crown's productions of loose hairs as natural 'combings.' Microscopic examination of the hair roots (recorded in photographs), showed signs of atrophy and fatty degeneration, and not that they had been forcibly pulled out. The jury was sufficiently confused to bring in a verdict of 'not proven'.[11]

Glaister's description of the scene of the crime, quoted above, is taken from his textbook, but the language, including the characteristic description of the 'soda-water-bottle-shaped marks of blood', was the same as in his official medical reports. Most of the textbook cases were in fact abbreviated versions of his reports: these, being official productions at the trial, had to be written in words that the jury could easily understand. Glaister then transposed the most interesting ones into his textbook without much rewriting.

In cases of this kind, and in many others during his subsequent work for the Crown, Glaister was not exercising any scientific skills other than careful and methodical observation. These were techniques which could be learned only from experience combined with study of the traditional methods of forensic medicine, as expounded by the experts of the past. The textbooks, such as Taylor's great compendium of cases, offered classic examples of deduction; and Glaister could illustrate them further from his own autopsies. The sensational reportage in the local press—particularly the *Weekly News* with its inventive line drawings—often made his work seem more mysterious and dramatic than it was.

This is well illustrated by one of his later cases, the Queen's Park murder.[12] Early in 1920, Albert Fraser and James Rollins, two men in their early twenties, committed a series of assaults and robberies: one would hold the victim while the other beat him and ripped out his pockets. The fourth assault ended in murder. Helen White, a young girl who lived with Fraser, acted as bait, and picked up a well-dressed man named Henry Senior in Hope Street. Followed by Fraser and Rollins, she took Senior by tram to Queen's Park recreation ground. They went into the shrubbery, where he was attacked, and died almost at once from rupture of the liver. His assailants, having ripped his trouser pockets, stole his coat and boots and pawned them; this led to their arrest about six days later, although they had fled to Belfast.[13]

Since Helen White gave evidence against Fraser and Rollins, the defence had little chance of maintaining their innocence, and concentrated on trying to reduce the charge from murder to culpable homicide, either by proving that the attack was a common affray which went wrong, or that Rollins was less to blame than Fraser. Glaister's post-mortem report showed that Senior had severe injuries in different places: there were marks of throttling around his neck; he had been hit in the face with a blunt instrument; and internal organs had been ruptured, either by a kick or with the knee of his attacker. Glaister concluded that Senior had been held and throttled by one assailant while the other hit him. His conclusions were based on straightforward reasoning. Senior had been violently throttled from behind, but this had not caused his death, which was due to internal injuries inflicted from in front; hence Glaister deduced two simultaneous attacks. Glaister's report confirmed the story of Helen White, who described how Senior had been pistol-whipped and kicked by Fraser while Rollins held him from behind with an arm round his neck: the defence counsel could not believe that the medical report was based on deduction alone, and asked several times whether Glaister had been told beforehand about White's evidence. Since Glaister had written his report before the two men were even caught, this suggestion was easily dismissed. Glaister also refuted the defence's suggestion that Fraser had used nothing more lethal than a fist—'I have been at this job for over thirty years, and I have formed some opinions as to what can be done with a fist.'[14] For good measure, he also found numerous bloodstains on the defendants' clothes. Both men were convicted and hanged. Glaister had used no techniques other than careful observations based on experience, but the defence's reaction enhanced his *mystique*.

It was through careful examination of the victim, the evidence, and the scene of the crime, that Glaister built his fearsome reputation as a medical jurist. That reputation also rested on his inimitable style and appearance in the courtroom.

> When the High Court comes round I am cock of the Walk,
> And discomfitted panels perspire in the dock,
> While I hold with the Judge an untechnical talk,
> For I've had 25 years of experience,
> And always refer to the penis as Cock.

His court style made Glaister a legendary figure. Over his 33 years as a medical jurist he developed his innate sense of theatre which both served the purpose of the prosecuting counsel and endeared Glaister to press and public. As a young man, he was dark-haired and wiry, of medium height, and with remarkably keen black eyes. Smoking thick black cheroots incessantly, he gave an impression of immense energy. In old age his hawk-like features, shiny bald head, vigorous moustache and small 'imperial' beard, together with his idiosyncratic retention of the Victorian style of silk hat, frock coat and wide Gladstonian collar, made him an unmistakable figure. Juries could not fail to be impressed, especially when, as often tended to happen later in his career, judges reminded them how distinguished he was.

Glaister worked during an era when the robust traditions of earlier times prevailed, and the law courts were still a legitimate piece of public entertainment, advertised in a way the public could not ignore. A month before the Circuit Court was due in Glasgow a warrant was issued to the Sheriff of Lanarkshire and his officers charging them with the duty of passing all the mercat crosses[15] in the Lanarkshire burghs to 'tell the people that the court is about to sit so that none may pretend ignorance.' Sheriffs' officers then left a copy of their declarations at each burgh cross.[16] Prisoners were arraigned eight days before their trials, and, if the case was of particular public interest, or unusually brutal or salacious, the courts printed handbills setting out the conditions of entry into the courtrooms. The public were forbidden to stand in the inner or outer passages of the courthouse, or to rise from their seats, or stand in the gallery. The side galleries were reserved for members of the Bar in wig and gown, and members of recognised legal societies. Opera glasses and cameras were forbidden, though as photographs of the accused in the dock sometimes appeared in the local press, this cannot have been well enforced. The circuit judges arrived with great ceremony: their pomp was somewhat reduced from the eighteenth-century days when they had walked for a mile through the streets to the sound of a solemn march played by the two elaborately dressed trumpeters who accompanied them on their travels, but even in the 1920s a 'fanfare of trumpets' preceded their entry into court. The representatives of the press took down the proceedings in shorthand, and the daily papers often carried the most sensational trials almost verbatim. In murder trials, large crowds of people who had not been able to get into the courtroom waited outside for news of the day's events. On such a stage, Glaister acted out his leading role.

Glaister, immensely self-confident, presented the medical evidence in lucid style and in layman's terms. Although he did not employ expressions quite as direct as those suggested in the *Ballad*, the 'untechnical talk' included such words as 'midriff', 'belly' and 'windpipe',[17] and left the jury in no doubt as to where the injuries were. His attitude towards cross-examining counsel was often daunting and sometimes taunting. One counsel, for example, attempted to draw him on the nature of the weapon allegedly used in a fatal stabbing. The defence claimed that as the point of the dagger was broken and the edges rather blunt, it could not have produced the stab wound. Glaister refuted this, and the following exchange occurred:

[Q] Could you cut a pencil or anything with it?
[A] It is not a very sharp weapon, not as sharp as a razor.
[Q] Could you even cut your finger on it? I am willing to try it.
[A] But will you allow me to stab you with it?[18]

In most cases, Glaister appeared for the prosecution, and his occasional appearances for the defence were mainly earlier in his career. It was always a temptation for a medico-legal expert who worked chiefly for the Crown to see his task as helping to secure a conviction. Unlike ordinary witnesses, the medical witness is permitted to give an opinion—on the cause of death for example—and does not have to confine himself to facts. An opinion is not a fact, but as the credibility of the forensic sciences improved, courts were naturally inclined to rely on the opinions of recognised medical experts. Like other great medical detectives, Glaister believed himself completely impartial in his evidence, but his reputation and sharp repartee had an obvious power to diminish the defence's case. One obituary noted that 'to some it might have appeared that his witness-bearing savoured somewhat of the advocate for the side to which he belonged.'[19]

Glaister, in the tradition of forensic medicine, taught his students that they must not be dogmatic in court when the evidence did not point to a straightforward conclusion; but once he had reached his own conclusion, he was unshakeable. To balance this account of his work for the prosecution, however, it should be remembered that his skills were also used to prevent prosecutions from taking place at all, or to have a charge reduced to a less serious one. If the prosecution pressed a case, Glaister did not always support it. In 1909, a young man named Joseph M'Clay was accused of murdering his wife after a quarrel which took place in bed. She hit him in the mouth and he caught her by the throat. The house showed no signs of violent struggle, and M'Clay gave himself up to the police. Glaister's report showed that Mrs M'Clay, who was in an advanced state of pulmonary tuberculosis, had died of heart failure, and not from asphyxiation. The prosecution, rather belatedly, reduced the charge during the trial from murder to culpable homicide, and after hearing evidence from the neighbours on Mrs M'Clay's bad habits, the judge sentenced M'Clay to two months' gaol.[20]

When Glaister believed himself right, he did not change his opinion, as can be seen in another trial for wife murder. This time the accused was an elderly man, alleged to have cut his wife's throat. The accused maintained that his wife had committed suicide, but Glaister was firmly of the opinion that the wound, which had been inflicted with a blunt kitchen knife, needed considerable force, and the angle was inconsistent with self-infliction:

> The position of the wound was such that the point of impact of a weapon in the hand of a right-handed person was too high to enable the striking hand to exercise sufficient force to produce a wound of the direction or depth found, and it would be difficult in performance, if not more difficult, in a left-handed person. Further, the blood-stains in the apartment indicated that the wound, however produced, had been made near the head of the bed—probably while the deceased was in bed—and it was extremely difficult to believe that after its infliction the deceased could have come out of bed and seated herself on the chair in the apartment.[21]

The medical witnesses for the defence nevertheless argued that suicide was theoretically possible, and as neighbours once again testified to the peaceable character of the accused, and to his wife's bad habits, he was acquitted. Glaister made up for defeat by devoting two pages of his *Textbook*, complete with photograph, to the case: reading his account, it is difficult to see how the defence succeeded.

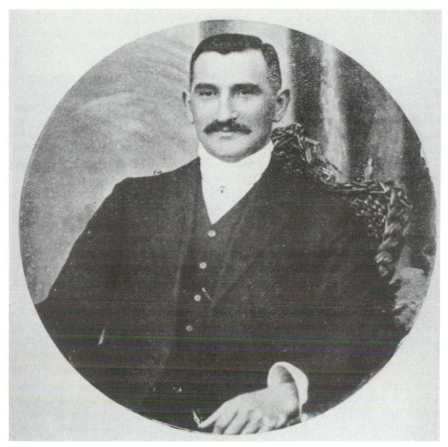

6   Oscar Slater (GUA)

Ironically, one of the cases which established Glaister's reputation is often seen as a gross miscarriage of justice, and although the details are well known, it cannot be omitted from any account of his career.[22] It also shows something of Glaister's characteristic obstinacy—a trait which he had in common with Spilsbury, Sydney Smith and other famous medical detectives of his time.

In 1909 Oscar Slater, a disreputable German Jew, was tried for murder. The victim was Marion Gilchrist, an 82-year old spinster, who lived in an elegant flat in the West End of Glasgow, and owned a valuable collection of jewellery. One evening her servant went out for a short time to buy a newspaper. A neighbour in the flat below heard strange sounds from Miss Gilchrist's flat, and went upstairs to knock on her door. The young servant girl returned at the same time, and they both encountered a man who came out of the flat and hurried down the stairs. The servant's apparent calm on seeing a strange man leave the flat, later gave many armchair detectives

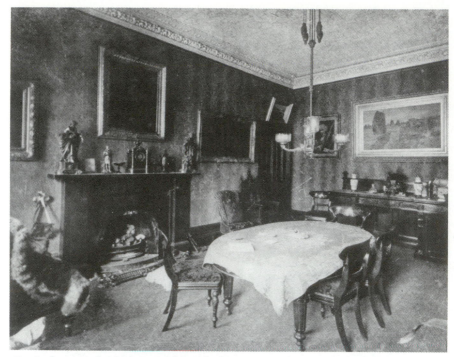

7   A photograph of Marion Gilchrist's dining room, for use in court. Her body was
found by the fireplace (GUA)

cause to argue that she must have known him. Marion Gilchrist was nervous
about admitting anyone when alone, and always kept the door locked: yet
the murderer had somehow gained an entrance. In the sitting room lay the
old lady, dead from head wounds inflicted with great brutality. Papers and
other objects in the bedroom were in disarray, but it was hard to say whether
anything had been taken.

Oscar Slater, who left for America with a mistress soon after the crime, was
linked to it only because he had sold a piece of jewellery, at first thought to be
Miss Gilchrist's, but conclusively proved to be his own property. He returned to
Britain voluntarily to stand trial. His alibi, that he was at home at the time
of the murder, came from his mistress and her servant, and was not believed.
He was convicted mainly on identification by Miss Gilchrist's servant and
another girl standing in the street, who claimed to have seen the escaping
murderer for a few seconds, and who was later shown to be thoroughly
unreliable. There was enough public disquiet to prevent his being hanged,
but he received a life sentence.

Slater's case divided the public like a smaller-scale Dreyfus affair: it aroused
xenophobia and anti-semitism and caused great alarm in Glasgow's large

Jewish community. In his summing up, the judge laid much stress on Slater's worthless character, though he had no record of violent behaviour. Although Slater the pimp was less heroic material than Dreyfus, Conan Doyle took the role of Zola in publicising Slater's plight;[23] after years of intermittent debate, Slater was finally released on license in 1927, and then grudgingly awarded a payment of £6,000 for wrongful conviction, a small recompense for nearly 20 years in prison.

The medical evidence rested entirely on the attempt to identify some stains on Slater's coat, and on the argument that a hammer in his possession might have been the murder weapon. Slater's hammer had a nine-inch shaft and a three-inch head: microscopic examination found signs of yellowish stains, which 'resembled red blood corpuscles of the mammalian type.'[24] The stains on the coat were similarly indeterminate. Both coat and hammer were said to have been washed, but more importantly, the medical witnesses for the Crown argued that the small hammer could have inflicted the appalling injuries on Marion Gilchrist—a point which Doyle and others disputed.[25] Given the lack of reliable direct evidence, circumstantial evidence of the type provided by Glaister was crucial in establishing some link between Slater and the victim.[26] It was not possible to conduct spectroscopic tests to establish whether the stains were mammalian blood, or even blood at all: and even if mammalian blood had been found, Glaister had, at that time, no way of establishing whether it was human blood. Yet when the judge asked Glaister; 'Suppose it were not a case of this kind, but some commercial question, how would you act?,' Glaister replied:

> If it were not a case of the kind it is, judging from my very long experience of examination of these stains, I would, without hesitation, say that, in my view, to the best of my knowledge and belief, they were red blood corpuscles.[27]

Glaister had a clear conscience about Slater's conviction. There was nothing erroneous in the medical evidence. It was *possible* that the hammer could inflict such wounds; the stains *might* be blood. Defence counsel made little effort to expose the weakness of this case. In the absence of more definite proof, the medical evidence should have counted for very little, but in the hysterical atmosphere surrounding the trial, Glaister's air of certainty doubtless influenced the jury. He included a lengthy summary of the evidence in his *Textbook*, under the heading 'multiple homicidal injuries', and there it remained until the fifth edition as an example to students of how to match injuries to a possible murder weapon. The case later provided more substantial instruction to police cadets in Glasgow as an example of how not to conduct a murder inquiry.

Unusual trials like Slater's may be remembered for years and increase the fame of the medical witnesses, but the bread-and-butter cases of Glaister's daily routine were of a different order. Murder committed for gain or passionate motives was a rare event: the average number of trials for murder in the whole of Scotland from the early twentieth century until the 1950s was around seven a year. Trials for infanticide in Scotland averaged about nine

per year in the first decade of the century, but had fallen to four by the
1930s. Drunken brawls produced most of the male subjects for Glaister's post-
mortems; drunken domestic arguments produced the female subjects. The
assailants were not charged with murder, but with culpable homicide, unless
the circumstances were particularly callous: there were about 34 charges of
culpable homicide a year in Scotland at the beginning of the century.[28] Like
infanticides, these trials often ended in a relatively light sentence. Such cases,
together with suicides and fatal accidents, provided Glaister with sufficient
material, though as he lost count of the autopsies he performed, the number
can only be conjectured.[29]

Nor were the murder weapons which Glaister examined particularly exotic.
He was well able to test for arsenic, antimony, and the other poisons detectable
at the time, but cases of this kind, as will be seen, were more likely to be
suicides or industrial accidents rather than murders. Firearms were sometimes
used, but the banal weapons for everyday crimes were usually boots or razors.
A survey of Glaister's cases gives the impression that there was scarcely a
domestic object which could not be used for violent purposes. Pokers, fire-
shovels, tools and cutlery were usually ready to hand: on one occasion the
newspapers described a fight in which two drunken women killed a third
with a poker, bottles and 'delf vessels'. Glaister's marginal note explains that
the 'vessels' were in fact the glazed ornaments familiar on Glasgow hearths
—two 'wally dugs'.[30]

Glaister's dual role as university professor and Crown witness meant that
many of the 'productions' to be exhibited in court came first to the university
to be tested. From that time until a decade ago, a miscellaneous collection of
objects was carried up the stairs to the department by relays of policemen. In
a murder trial, Glaister might conduct tests for blood and other matter on
seventy or more productions. Clothing, the most common production, could
at least be transported easily and took up little space, but many larger items
such as three-piece suites, industrial equipment, gates, fences, and rolls of
linoleum had also to be accommodated. Glaister often worked late into the
night testing productions, not only in the laboratory, but behind his town
house in a converted stable.

Glaister's fame, like that of Spilsbury, rests on his work as a medical
detective, rather than major contributions to forensic science. Indeed, it is
hard to see how so busy a man, working entirely on his own in the earlier
years, could have found time for extensive researches, which were more easily
carried out in the larger medico-legal institutes of Europe, notably in Vienna.
Glaister refused even to employ a secretary to type out his medical reports;
he typed them himself from the longhand drafts he wrote in unused university
examination books under the familiar injunction *candidates are warned that
marks may be lost by illegible writing*. In any case, the most notable contributions to forensic science at the time were coming from chemists and
biologists, particularly in the field of serology. The great medical detectives,
like the great surgeons, demonstrated a mastery of technique rather than an
ability for original research; but like the surgeons, they needed to keep abreast
of any scientific discoveries relevant to their work.

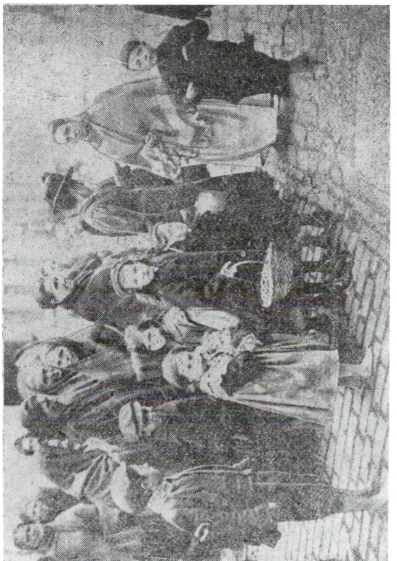

8 A crowd gathers outside a house where a murder has taken place in the Calton district, 1911. Much of Glaister's work was conducted against this kind of background (GP)

Yet it would be wrong to see Glaister purely as a masterly interpreter of other men's discoveries; he published some valuable work which made effective use of his experience in both forensic medicine and public health. Arsenical poisoning, although rare, was a subject which stirred the public imagination because of a number of sensational murder trials in the past, but Glaister treated it as an industrial problem. He was a medical referee under the Workmen's Compensation Act, investigating claims for compensation in industrial injuries; and his work on arsenical poisoning had practical significance.

Around 1900 Glaister was called as a consultant to see a dying labourer. The man, an employee of the local bleachworks, was jaundiced, and post-mortem examination showed characteristic signs of the destruction of red blood corpuscles. The patient had been taken ill after climbing into a large retort to clean it: the retort contained the detritus of several weeks of bleach production—a mixture of manganese chloride, manganese dioxide and hydrochloric acid. Glaister knew that the hydrochloric acid was produced in the bleachworks, and that it was made from Spanish pyrites which contained, amongst other things, arsenic. During the process of manufacture, the arsenic remained in the industrial debris in the form of arsenic acid: the workman had used an iron shovel and zinc-galvanised iron pail to clean out the debris, and this had produced a chemical reaction which led to his being poisoned by arseniuretted hydrogen. Chemical experiments with the debris produced the noxious gas which, as Glaister remarked, resulted from the workman himself unconsciously setting off Marsh's process for isolating arsenic.[31]

The implications for improved industrial practice moved Glaister to search for all available information on arsene gas poisoning, and in 1908 he published a book entitled *Poisoning by Arseniuretted Hydrogen or Hydrogen Arsenide*. In collecting information from many different sources, Glaister released the subject from 'the limbo of rarities for which information had to be sought among the isolated case records.'[32] He was able to trace 121 cases of illness or deaths among a disparate group of victims including medico-legists conducting the Marsh test, military balloonists inhaling impure hydrogen, workers engaged in the production of aniline dyes and bleaching powder, and householders lingering too long amongst arsenical flock wallpaper from which gas was released by the action of mould.[33]

> If your wife take a drug with intent to abort,
> It's cases like these I hold as my forte,
> And I furnish a medicolegal report,
> In terms of Vic.2, Cap.3, Section 10.
> With details that necessitate clearing the court.

Although the investigation of violent death brought Glaister into the public eye, his medico-legal work was very wide-ranging. As in his early career of police surgeon, he conducted clinical examinations in cases of rape, child molestation, homosexuality and the like. This side of his work, however, had little publicity except amongst medical students. Courts were often cleared in these cases, and the press did not report them. Reticence persisted throughout the inter-war years, and may contribute to the illusion that certain forms of behaviour are typical only of the late twentieth century. Glasgow's High Court was divided into two: the north court heard all the more printable forms of serious crime, while the south court, known familiarly to the crime reporters as 'the dirty court', often went unreported.[34] Glaister appeared in both.

Another regular task for the complete medical detective was clinical assessment of a defendant's fitness to plead. During the nineteenth century, the study of insanity became a specialised branch of medicine, and psychiatric doctors made strong claims to be summoned as experts in criminal cases where the defendant's capacity was in doubt.[35] By the later nineteenth century, the defence usually called a specialist when arguing that the defendant was mentally unbalanced, but the Crown still used forensic experts like Glaister. Hence Glaister found himself against weighty colleagues such as D K Henderson, lecturer in psychological medicine at the university, or Ivy McKenzie, a distinguished pathologist with a special interest in psychiatry. Glaister's psychiatric reports were based on interviews with the prisoner, and sometimes with his family. A survey of Western Circuit records suggests that Glaister rarely found the prisoners unfit to plead, even in cases which his colleagues automatically assumed to demonstrate unsound mind, such as unmarried mothers who drowned their babies in the Clyde.[36] Gilbert Garrey, physician to the Duke Street prison, regularly contradicted Glaister's opinion, and found prisoners unfit to plead. When Glaister did detect unsoundness of mind, the prosecution invariably accepted his judgment. He continued with this work after his retirement from the chair, until a few months before his death in 1932. It should be remarked, however, that Glaister's reluctance to detect unsound mind was not necessarily against the interests of the defendant, except in charges which carried the death penalty. Those found unfit to plead were given an indefinite custodial sentence in an institution: after the Mental Deficiency Act of 1913, such custody might be a life-sentence, even though the degree of mental deficiency was slight. Finding the prisoner fit to plead might, if there were mitigating circumstances, result in a short gaol term.

Glaister's tough views on insanity once had an odd result, as he recorded in a carefully-worded account in his textbook. In 1903 William Purves, a middle-aged river pilot, earning a comfortable salary of between £400 and £600 a year, quarrelled with his wife because she insisted on attending spiritualist meetings late into the night against his wishes. The wife refused to share his bedroom, and called in two doctors to investigate his sanity. Purves, thinking they had been called in to consult on his personal problems, allowed them to examine him and discussed his domestic relations with them. He was later committed to Gartnavel asylum and remained there four months until his lawyers obtained his release by calling in Glaister and another doctor to examine him. In Glaister's view, Purves was not dangerous. On leaving the asylum, Purves found himself unemployed, as his employers refused to take him back, and he raised an action for damages against the doctors who had certified him. He failed in two lengthy lawsuits. In 1907, having no money left, and driven by an acute desire to 'ventilate his wrongs', he took a revolver and fired three bullets into the thigh of the senior certifying doctor. At his trial, Purves refused to plead insanity, even though he had again been judged insane by two further doctors after his arrest. An unusual legal situation arose, in which the prosecution was prepared to accept a plea of insanity, but the defendant would not offer it. The unfortunate pilot, who insisted that he had every good reason to shoot the doctor, and knew exactly what he was doing, was sentenced to seven years' penal servitude.[37]

Glaister, as men in his profession must, shielded himself from morbid speculations, and was able to detach himself completely from his work when not engaged in it.[38] He seems to have been helped by his strong religious convictions (he was a Congregationalist), overlaid by his belief in the then fashionable theory of eugenics, or, as he called it, 'social bionomics'. Eugenics provided a convenient framework for explaining both crime and squalor: the two strands of the medical police tradition. Glaister argued that in the slum districts of Glasgow, crime, drunkenness, uncleanliness, overcrowding and high infant mortality rates sprang from the same root: moral inadequacy amongst the poor. He subscribed to the views of the Poor Law Commission of 1909 that the 'degenerate' and incapable, the feeble-minded and the incorrigibly idle, should be removed from the community as criminals were, while the more tractable should be vigorously instructed in hygiene and given severe penalties if they neglected their children.[39] James Burn Russell, Glasgow's Medical Officer of Health, who attended the same church as Glaister, produced a famous statistical correlation between ill-health and over-crowding in Glasgow's notorious 'single-end' housing.[40] Glaister inverted Russell's judgment that poor housing was the source of many of Glasgow's ills, and argued instead that low moral fibre caused the inhabitants to tolerate poor housing and its attendant evils.[41] Glaister believed that the authorities could enforce individual hygiene and morality to solve the city's problems. Such certainties may have supported him in his journeys through Glasgow's lower depths.

At the end of the war, therefore, Glaister contemplated the prospect of heading a department which should be entirely devoted to forensic medicine. In 1919, before the division between public health and forensic medicine took place, a new assistant joined him. This was his second son, then aged 27, the youngest of his six children. Glaister always referred formally to his son as 'John Glaister, Junior', but the Glasgow medical world inevitably dubbed them 'Old John' and 'Young John'. The younger Glaister had taken his degree at Glasgow and learned forensic medicine in his father's classes; until 1928 they worked together. Although, as will be seen, the younger Glaister inherited much of his father's manner and style, their collaboration signalled a change in the nature of forensic medicine in the university: it began a period of transition from the days of the single-handed medical detective to the group effort of the modern scientific department.

CHAPTER FOUR

The 1920s: Blood, Hair and Gunshots

Dynasties are common in the medical profession, and there were excellent financial reasons for them in the days before the National Health Service, when a son would assist, and then succeed, his father in the family practice. Scottish academic life was also somewhat inbred, with many professors coming from professorial families.[1] The Glaisters had a nearby example to follow: in Edinburgh, the Regius Professor of Forensic Medicine, Sir Henry Littlejohn, was succeeded in 1906 by his son Harvey. The younger generation of Glaisters was firmly entrenched in the medical world: both sons became doctors, and three of the daughters married medical men.

'Young John' did not plan this career, for he had no early interest in medicine. Born into much greater affluence than his father, he was idle at school, and his main ambition was to be an actor in musical comedy. His autobiography tells of the interview in which he confessed this hope to his father. The elder Glaister, himself well regarded as a domestic singer and piano player, responded in two words: 'Forget it.' The son tried another suggestion:

If the stage wouldn't or couldn't have me, then a barrister I would be—I had formed the impression, still unbroken, that a certain histrionic ability was one of the hallmarks of a successful courtroom personality.[2]

The elder Glaister compromised, suggesting law studies after a medical degree: in fact the son later qualified as a barrister, but by that time the law was only a useful supplement to a career in forensic medicine. Theatrical flair, however, was to serve him well, as it had his father.

In 1916, as soon as he qualified in medicine, young Glaister joined the army. He served in Palestine, where he treated Turkish prisoners in the emergency hospitals, under atrocious conditions. The mortality rate was appalling. After dealing with an epidemic of typhus, he succumbed to bacillary dystentery, followed by influenza, and returned home in the last months of the war emaciated beyond recognition. His experiences left him with permanent health problems and a fear, noticed by several of his contemporaries, lest he contract infection through his work. Although he mastered this anxiety, his precautions when conducting a post-mortem were always highly elaborate.

53

During the war he married Jean, daughter of the Town Clerk of Glasgow, Sir John Lindsay. Husband and wife had the excellent social connections which would have enabled him to embark on a successful private practice, but he was now determined to build a career in forensic medicine. Like his father's, his private practice was short-lived, and for some years he supported himself with a variety of part-time posts, supplementing the modest pay as his father's assistant with fees for medico-legal examinations. His family connections probably helped to secure him work with Glasgow Corporation, to which he was medico-legal adviser and examiner; and he lectured to the police on medical jurisprudence. He also deputised for his father as medical referee under the Cremation Act of 1902: cremation, then regarded as rather eccentric, required stricter medical certification than burial. The elder Glaister was an early supporter of cremation, as his interest in public health made him sensitive to Glasgow's overcrowded graveyards. Both Glaisters were referees for the Maryhill crematorium, which was run by the Cremation and Burial Reform Society; the doctors' duty was to check for irregularities in the death certificates before cremation could take place.

Young Glaister's most important work at this time was in his father's laboratory, carrying out chemical and microscopic tests. As the 1920s went on, he occasionally appeared as second medical examiner in post mortems, and supplemented his father's evidence in court. The position here was delicate. The chief medical examiner for the Crown has to call a second doctor to assist him in serious cases; by the early 1920s the elder Glaister was working regularly with John Anderson, pathologist at the Victoria infirmary, and sometimes with his former university assistant, Andrew Allison, now a police surgeon, who was lecturing in forensic medicine at St Mungo's. To supplant these experienced men with his own son would have upset the unwritten protocol of medico-legal examinations, especially as the fees for Crown work were the subject of polite, but intense, interest to those qualified to earn them.

Acting as his father's 'back-room boy,' the younger Glaister found a niche in the medico-legal world by developing research interests where he was recognised as the expert. He could also keep his busy father abreast of new techniques in forensic science. When 'Old John' was appointed, professors were not expected to distinguish themselves in research,[3] but the war encouraged a great expansion of research in both science and medicine. The German example of university staff with a strong research commitment was becoming more compelling in Britain. In the 1920s, forensic science began to move away from the wide-ranging expertise of the elder Glaister, into more detailed and specialised studies. The younger Glaister became particularly interested in two of them: hairs and blood.

Forensic scientists need to adapt new ideas in basic science to their own purposes: discoveries in physics, chemistry or biology may have legal significance which needs to be tested comprehensively in the laboratory. There will be a time-lag between the discovery of a new scientific technique and its acceptance in the courts. Occasional laboratory errors which would not invalidate scientific results are unacceptable to the law: forensic scientists have to convince the courts that their methods allow of no mistakes. As scientific techniques become more exact, the time-lag between a discovery and its acceptance in law has shortened, but the 1920s were a difficult period. A number of important new methods were available, but their acceptance was slow, both because of the possibility of laboratory errors and the ill-informed attitudes of some members of the legal profession. The Glaisters found themselves in the front line in persuading Scottish courts to accept new ideas, particularly in the changing techniques for the identification of bloodstains.

In the Oscar Slater case, the elder Glaister invited criticism by sounding more positive about blood testing in court than was proper, although his written report was suitably cautious. He could identify a suspicious stain only as mammalian blood; he could not distinguish the blood of man from other mammals. It was usual to conduct several tests for blood. In fresh stains, microscopic examination might reveal blood corpuscles; old stains had to be soaked in saline solution and subjected to several chemical tests, the most useful of which produced haemin crystals visible under the microscope. The spectroscopic test could identify very small stains: here prisms in the microscope broke down the colouring matter of blood into characteristic bands of colours from the spectrum, and the variations also gave some idea of the bloodstain's age.[4] All this painstaking work could easily go for nothing if the defence offered an innocent explanation for an incriminating bloodstain—that it was animal blood, or not the blood of the victim.

In the late 1890s, Rudolf Kraus in Vienna reported on the 'precipitin test', and his results were rapidly elaborated by several European scientists. If a rabbit were injected with blood serum from another animal, its own blood reacted defensively to produce an antiserum. Antiserum taken from the rabbit would then produce a precipitate if mixed with serum from the other animal. In 1901, P Uhlenhuth confirmed the forensic importance of this test by showing how specific it was: he injected rabbits with human blood and tested the antiserum on 19 different types of animal blood: only human blood reacted positively.[5] Uhlenhuth was also able to identify human blood on all kinds of bloodstained articles. Shortly afterward, G H F Nuttall in Cambridge exposed some of the drawbacks of the test: groups of related animals would produce a certain amount of precipitate in the rabbit's antiserum, and a series of tests was necessary to eliminate this factor.[6]

Forensic laboratories all over the world had an obvious interest in confirming such research, but the processes were intricate, expensive, and time-consuming. If any impurities contaminated the serum the test might fail, and elaborate controls were necessary to check its accuracy.

By 1910 the Prussian courts were accepting the validity of the precipitin test, but the British were more cautious. The Royal Institute of Public Health was carrying out experiments in London,[7] and the Home Office consulted Sir

William Willcox, one of the leading forensic pathologists of the day. In 1907 Willcox would not use the test to say more than that there was a 'presumption' of human blood: by 1910, if he had obtained a well-marked reaction in the test, combined with positive results in the other standard tests, he was prepared to use it in court.[8] Anti-serum took up to two months to make, and commercial supplies were not easy to obtain: the Germans seemed to be cornering the market, which was then disrupted by war.

In Glasgow, the elder Glaister was also cautious. In 1922 a reviewer in the *Glasgow Medical Journal* took him to task for being behind the times in the fourth edition of his textbook, which had appeared the previous year. Glaister described the test in detail, but repeated the conclusion from his earlier editions that the medical witness still could not answer the question 'Is the blood that of a human being?'[9] His critic commented:

> It is now many years since the precipitin test was proved capable of answering the question and unless the medical witness has up-to-date knowledge he will become, as the Professor says of the voluble witness 'a Godsend to the opposing counsel with a weak case.' [10]

The younger Glaister remedied this deficiency by making a special study of the forensic applications of the precipitin test for his MD thesis.[11] He concentrated on making the test more accurate, and on methods of identifying bloodstains at various ages and in very small quantities. He also described what happened when bloodstains were washed in in different ways. He found that he could use the test successfully on one thirty-second of a drop of blood; soap invalidated the test, but water did not.[12] By the mid 1920s both Glaisters were experienced in the latest techniques, though the resources of their laboratory were not enough to provide regular supplies of anti-serum, and they had to import it from Dresden. Young Glaister was then called as assistant doctor in cases where the test was important.

At first, defence counsel did not seriously challenge the test, as it was not always a crucial part of the evidence.

In January 1922, the body of Elizabeth Benjamin, a Jewish girl aged 14, was found in the back green of a tenement in Whiteinch. The girl's father sold drapery on the credit system in the tenements, but as he was ill, his daughter had been going his rounds and collecting payments from his usual customers. When her body was found, the wrists were tied, and there were several head wounds. Blood on the stair and doorstep of a neighbouring tenement house led to the arrest of a married couple, William and Helen Harkness.

Professor Glaister and Anderson carried out the post mortem and found that, although the girl had been stunned by blows to the head from a sharp instrument, death was due to suffocation from a handkerchief rolled up and stuffed down her throat. Her wrists had been tied after death so that her body could be lifted and hidden in the wash-house before it was moved to the back green. Seventy articles arrived at the forensic medicine department for examination, including the clothing of victim and accused, a steel reamer—

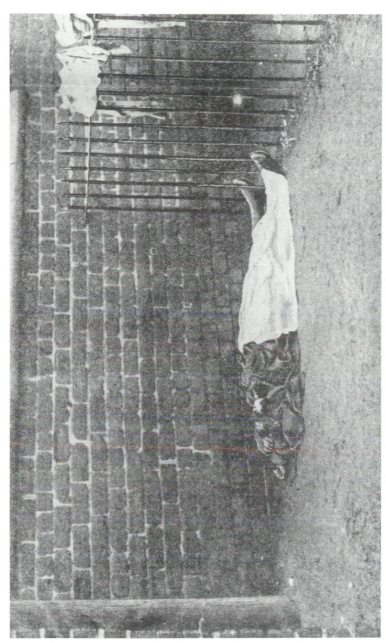

9   The body of Elizabeth Benjamin in the back-court at Whiteinch (GP)

a pointed tool used by Harkness in his trade as a riveter—a chair, a doormat, linoleum, a piece of the skirting board, four pieces of wallpaper and part of the casing from the wash-house boiler.[13]

In the laboratory, the Glaisters found extensive staining from mammalian blood on the Harkness clothes and furniture, and on the reamer. They carried out the precipitin test on four productions, including wallpaper, where there were large blood clots, since at that time they could use the test only on fairly large stains. The elder Glaister dealt summarily with the defence's suggestion that the handkerchief could have accidentally lodged in the girl's throat during an attempt to gag her, and fended off some ill-prepared criticisms of the precipitin test:

> Unless you get a sufficient quantity of blood you cannot make the test with certainty. In the case of the four instances I have mentioned we had sufficient blood to enable us to make the test without doubt.[14]

The defence did not press the issue, and the judge accepted Glaister's findings in his summing up. But although Glaister's evidence was important in establishing the fact of murder, the blood tests were not as crucial for the prosecution as the evidence of William Harkness's brother, who had helped him move the body from the wash-house. The motive for the murder was the money which Elizabeth Benjamin had collected—£2 in all. The Harknesses considered it hardly worth the effort, as Mrs Harkness remarked to her brother-in-law: 'it was the factoress [rent collector] they meant—they would have got about £50.'[15] Both were sentenced to death: William Harkness was hung and his wife reprieved to life imprisonment.

The Glaisters again used the precipitin test without incident in another trial in 1925. John Keen and three other men were accused of stabbing a Bengali pedlar, Noor Mohamed. Mohamed lived in a tenement in Port Dundas with several other Bengali immigrants; his brother Nathoo, who had married a local girl, lived in the next tenement. The small group of Indians, several of whom had served in the army during the war, were exotic aliens in the back streets; they lived quietly, however, and police and other witnesses were adamant that there was no racial feeling against them. One evening, Keen and two others came to Nathoo's house and there was an argument over some goods they wanted to take. Nathoo ran to his brother's house, while Keen got together a gang which attacked the Bengalis: Noor Mohamed was dragged out and stabbed. The Glaisters identified human blood on the clothing of two of the defendants, and on Keen's boots.[16]

Representing one of Keen's associates was the formidable Craigie Aitchison, later Lord Advocate under the second Labour government. In the Keen case, the defence did not challenge the precipitin test, but tried to upset Professor Glaister's evidence over the age of the bloodstains. It was essential for the prosecution to prove that the stains were recent when tested, and Glaister was able to prove this because corpuscles were still visible under the microscope.[17] Again the precipitin test was not a crucial part of the outcome. The knife

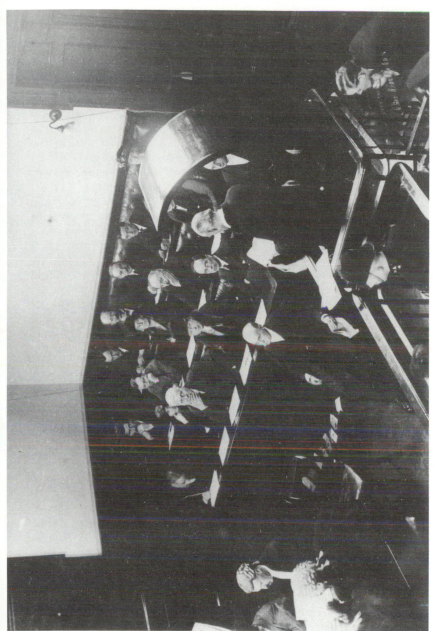

10   John Glaister Sr reading his medical report in the Harkness trial. This is a rare photograph of a trial in session: the jury is facing Glaister with several labelled productions lying on the floor in front of them. The broom leaning against the door is also part of the evidence (*The Bulletin*)

which had stabbed Noor Mohamed could be traced back to Keen, and he alone was clearly identified by eyewitnesses. He was found guilty of murder, and hung.[18]

In 1926 Aitchison threw the whole issue of precipitin testing in Scottish courts into confusion, for he had spotted Glaister's weak point. The trial was that of an itinerant basket maker, who was accused of assaulting and strangling a four-year-old girl in Stirling. There was a second charge of sexual assault on another little girl on the same night. The back courts behind the Stirling houses were a hazardous maze after dark, and the child's body was not found until after several hours of frantic searching by family and neighbours: feelings were so high in Stirling that an innocent stranger was nearly lynched by a crowd of women. The accused had been seen in the neighbourhood, and was already known to the police. He was described by several children, who recognised him by his shock of yellow hair, and he was further recognisable by clawlike fingers, deformed in an accident.

The attack was so brutal that it disturbed even Glaister's professional calm. 'Professor Glaister is not usually given to garnishing his reports with adjectives,' commented the judge, on hearing the medical report's description of the 'inhuman force' which had been used.[19] The murder had taken place in 1924, but the case was delayed over legal technicalities, including the question of the defendant's sanity, since he had frequently been in mental hospitals.

At the first hearing, the man was committed to an asylum, in spite of the elder Glaister's characteristic decision that he was fit to plead though of 'a somewhat demented' character.[20] After some months, he was declared sane, released, and re-arrested. The elder Glaister had found bloodstains under the defendant's nails, on his clothes and a towel he had used for washing shortly after the murder: three months later, both Glaisters identified the blood on the clothing and towel as human, their tests having been delayed while they waited for anti-serum from Dresden. The stains were important to the defence, since the accused claimed to have helped with a calving, and that the stains were cow's blood.

Aitchison and Professor Glaister were old adversaries, and well used to each other's court style. As a defence counsel, Aitchison took care to be well-informed on medical evidence, and frequently put medical witnesses through long cross-examinations, questioning the accuracy of their methods at all points.[21] In this trial, Aitchison led Glaister through the whole medical report, implying that Glaister had not carried out enough of the conventional tests for blood, and that the delay before the precipitin tests invalidated the results. Both of these arguments Glaister firmly rejected, believing that his son's work had confirmed previous suggestions that the precipitin test would work even with very old stains. Aitchison, according to legal custom, quoted from a number of textbooks, including Glaister's own second edition. 'You should get the fourth,' commented Glaister.[22] Aitchison *had* got the fourth, and opened it at the damaging page where Glaister stated that forensic science was not sufficiently advanced to allow the medical expert to determine the age of a stain, nor whether it was human blood. He read out Glaister's own words of five years previously and asked, 'Do you agree with that?' Glaister replied,

> No. I think you will find in the next edition that I will be able to answer each of these questions in a different way. When I wrote that that was my belief, but we can from long experience not only form an opinion as to age, but we can form an opinion as to the source of the blood from the body and also which class of animal to which it belongs.[23]

Aichison continued to press Glaister on whether the tests had been made too long after the murder, but Glaister would not be moved:

> We have taken blood as far back as 15 years and we have been able to find the serum and find a positive reaction to human blood.

'Would you hang a man on that?' asked Aitchison improperly, and Glaister responded, 'That is not for me to say.'[24] Young Glaister was also called, and had to side-step Aitchison's insinuation that he alone was the expert and his father's evidence incompetent.[25]

Aitchison convinced judge and jury that the precipitin test was unreliable, and Lord Alness commented in his summing up:

> We have the dogmatic statement in Professor Glaister's 1921 edition of his textbook that there is no use in trying to establish the difference in human from mammalian blood. Yet in 1925 he states that this is possible. There is no evidence given for this change of mind, perhaps the advance of medical science.[26]

The jury took only 30 minutes to find a verdict of not proven on the murder charge, but found the accused guilty of indecent assault against the other child, and he received a four-year sentence. Aitchison retained his reputation for never having a client found guilty of murder.[27]

But even before Glaister's next edition came out in 1931, the courts were accepting the precipitin test as standard practice. In 1927 James M'Kay was tried for the murder of his mother, Agnes Arbuckle, in a case popularly known as 'the Body in the Bunker'. Mrs Arbuckle's head and some other parts of her body, burned in places, were found on the bank of the Clyde. Her son was charged with murder, and directed the police to the coal bunker in her house, where the rest of the body was hidden. M'Kay was destitute, but had taken out a £15 insurance policy on his mother's life; after her death he sold virtually everything in the house, and was practising her signature in order to obtain her nest egg of £83 from the bank. The defence had to admit that M'Kay dismembered his mother, but argued that she had died of natural causes and fallen into the fire; when her son came home he tried to get rid of the body to avert suspicion from himself and to get hold of the money.[28] Much depended on whether the defence could plausibly argue that the wounds on the body were not the cause of death, but the result of clumsy dissection.

Mrs Arbuckle's body was a textbook case in which to exhibit the art of the forensic pathologist. Professor Glaister, who carried out the post mortem with John Anderson, was adamant that the wounds had been inflicted before death, since gaping wounds of that type could not be produced in a dead body. In spite of its time in the river, the hair held blood clots which could only have come from a living person. The burns on the body, which showed no blistering, were also characteristic of burns some time after death, probably from an attempt to prevent identification.[29] Glaister and Anderson searched the house carefully for bloodstains, but since they found very little, Glaister concluded that it had been carefully washed. The defence asked, 'Is that a suspicion that you formed because you did not find the blood you hoped to find?' Glaister replied with his usual aplomb, 'No. I did not hope to find it. I take what the King sends me, no more and no less.'[30] Human blood, however, was found on the underside of a cleaned chair, suggesting that it had spurted from wounds in a living person. Glaister carried out the precipitin test, and found evidence of human blood on M'Kay's clothes and on a saw; the defence did not dispute this. Acceptance of the test had now progressed so far that defence counsel asked Glaister why he had not used it on all the stained items. Glaister's answer was that the cost of the test was so high that he could only take samples.[31] M'Kay was hung, largely on forensic evidence which mixed traditional techniques of close observation of the body with the latest scientific methods. By this time, serology was moving on, and the courts would soon have to cope not only with the implications of distinguishing human from animal blood, but the question of human blood groups.

Meanwhile, the younger Glaister developed his second research interest, the study of hairs and fibres. This was one of many lines of research followed by forensic scientists in the 1920s. Forensic science, as he described it, was concerned with 'the key of interchange'—the evidence which a criminal unwittingly left behind, or took away with him.[32] The interchange could take many forms: biological interchange might include blood, semen, hair, body tissues, and so forth: other types of interchange could include anything from a bullet to a fragment of glass.

In the inter-war period, most of the developments in forensic medicine were negative tests, that is, they served mainly to *exclude* a person from suspicion. Blood testing, whether for human blood or, later, for the type of blood, could be used to prove innocence, but not guilt, since many individuals shared the same blood type. When it was realised that blood types were hereditary, blood types could also be used to disprove, but not prove, paternity.[33] The only conclusive evidence of biological individuality was the fingerprint, but the careful criminal would not leave one. All such forensic work was based on statistical probabilities: in the case of fingerprints, the probability of two people having the same prints was infinitesimal.

The only other forensic study to approach a high degree of certainty in the 1920s was ballistics, where great skill was exercised in identifying spent bullets by the characteristic markings from the rifle barrel which fired them.[34] Biological tests were not nearly as advanced, but the search continued for a test which should be as precise as a fingerprint. Hairs, with their great variety, seemed a possibility, and Glaister spent much time, as he said, 'splitting hairs' for his D.Sc. thesis, submitted in 1927.[35]

This was painstaking work, leading Glaister to search through zoos and museums for the hairs of mammals, and to find ways of comparing them with each other and with hairs from the different races of man. Glaister shared his father's passion for photography, and made photo-micrographs of hairs cut horizontally and vertically. He elaborated on earlier studies which showed that the central section (medulla) of hairs was characteristic for each type of animal, and by exhaustive comparison he was able to distinguish between hairs from the outer fur and woolly under-pelt of animals.[36]

The fruit of this laborious work was published a few years later by the Egyptian government, together with an Atlas of some 1700 photographs.[37] It was well received by forensic specialists, though criticised for lacking an index, and Glaister appealed to historical interests by showing that the structure of hair on Egyptian mummies had been virtually unaltered by time. His work was mainly useful for assisting with the classification of hair from different mammals, different races, and different parts of the body. Although hairs have individual characteristics, hairs from the same head vary enormously, and it has not yet proved possible to trace a hair to its owner with the certainty of a fingerprint. For forensic purposes however, knowledge of hairs could be of value in building up a case, especially if they were cut, dyed, or waved in a peculiar way. Glaister became an expert on such identification.

Hairs were frequently cited as evidence in murder trials, but were used mainly to strengthen other evidence. In 1926, an attendant at Dykebar mental hospital, near Paisley, was accused of raping and murdering a nurse, his fellow-worker, in a field near the hospital. Her head had been repeatedly banged against a stone in the ground. Preciptin tests showed human blood-stains on his clothing, and further evidence came from pubic hair, similar to the nurse's, caught in the fly-front of his trousers.[38] The accused made little effort to deny the charges, and Craigie Aitchison's defence concentrated on his state of mind: the sentence was 15 years for culpable homicide.

Hairs could be conclusive if they appeared in unlikely places. In 1924, James Thomson was charged with having stolen the contents of a parked car in Maybole. He made off with a rug, two furs, a scarf, 35s. in cash, two loaves, a sponge cake, six eggs and half a pound of butter. On being chased, he not surprisingly dropped his booty and ran home. None of the witnesses had seen him clearly, but on his sleeve the Glaisters found an unusual mixture of black skunk fur and fibres of light brown wool like those of the rug. He was sentenced to 18 months.[39]

By the mid 1920s, the younger Glaister was developing a reputation in his own right, though inevitably overshadowed by his father's courtroom fame. In 1928, at the age of 36, he branched out on his own taking up the chair of forensic medicine at the University of Cairo. This appointment followed an upheaval in the highly specialised circles of Scottish forensic medicine. In

1927 Harvey Littlejohn, the Regius Professor at Edinburgh, died. His post was sought by both the younger Glaister and Sydney Smith, Littlejohn's protégé, at that time professor of forensic medicine in Cairo and chief medico-legal examiner to the British administration in Egypt. Glaister offered numerous influential testimonials, including a frigidly impersonal one from his father,[40] but Smith, nine years his senior, and with ten years of experience in Egypt, was successful. Smith replaced Littlejohn in Edinburgh and Glaister replaced Smith in Cairo, though in a post newly under the control of an Egyptian administration. Smith was convinced that Littlejohn's death, the immediate cause of these manoeuvres, had been hastened by worry over the Merrett case, in which not only Littlejohn, but Smith himself and both the Glaisters, took part.[41]

Although the murder of Bertha Merrett did not require the use of novel techniques in forensic medicine, it stimulated the public imagination because of the unusual circumstances, and because of the notable confrontation between the Scottish forensic pathologists for the prosecution, and Sir Bernard Spilsbury for the defence.[42]

The events of this well-known case can be briefly recalled. In March 1926, Mrs Merrett was shot in the head as she sat at a desk in her Edinburgh house. The bullet, from a very small pistol, entered behind her right earhole, and passed forward for about an inch through the bony structures of the skull, without damaging the brain. She died of meningitis in the Royal Infirmary a fortnight later, and although sometimes conscious, seemed to have little idea of what had happened. Her son, Donald, had been in the room with her: their daily maid was cleaning in the next room, but was incoherent about what had occurred. In one statement she claimed to have seen the pistol falling from Mrs Merrett's hand, in another, she had not. The police found the gun, belonging to Donald Merrett, on the floor, but made no effort to trace the cartridge. Mrs Merrett was a widow of blameless character and in comfortable circumstances. Her son, a student, was only 17, and there seemed no motive for murder. The police therefore charged the semi-conscious Mrs Merrett with attempted suicide,[43] but, as she was in a dangerous condition, no-one discussed the circumstances with her. Harvey Littlejohn wrote a perfunctory post-mortem report which he later had cause to regret, stating that

> 'There was nothing to indicate the distance at which the discharge of the weapon took place, whether from a few inches or a greater distance. So far as the position of the wound is concerned, the case is consistent with suicide.'[44]

A few months later, the police discovered that Donald Merrett had been leading a dissipated life, and that he had systematically forged his mother's signature on cheques before her death. Further evidence came from the doctor who first examined Mrs Merrett, that the wound showed none of the powder blackening expected if the gun had been fired close to her head in the usual manner of suicides. Nurses and relatives also reported that she had made confused comments which implicated her son. Merrett was tried for murder, but Aitchison, for the defence, had the great advantage of the incompetent behaviour of the police and Littlejohn's original suggestion of suicide.

Mrs Merrett died in April 1926. During the summer the police reopened the case, and Littlejohn began to reconsider his report. He sought the advice of Sydney Smith, then in Edinburgh on vacation from Cairo, who had a particular interest in ballistics and gunshot wounds. Smith was perturbed by the improbability of the angle of the wound and the absence of powder blackening, and recommended that experiments be made.[45] In November, both the prosecution and the defence asked Professor Glaister for his assistance. He refused to be a defence witness, but the Glaisters went to Edinburgh to carry out tests with Littlejohn. The aim of the tests was to duplicate the effects of the pistol shot, and to see the effects on skin of shots fired at various distances. Littlejohn and the Glaisters carried out the tests with the pistol which had killed Mrs Merrett, and with the same type of ammunition. They tested the effects on white cardboard, but for extra realism they used a freshly amputated leg from the victim of a railway accident, though the prosecution decided to spare the jury these details.[46] Littlejohn and Glaister wrote separate reports, both affirming that suicide was most unlikely because of the absence of powder blackening around the wound. Littlejohn's report did not mention the experiment on the leg; Glaister's referred briefly to 'further experiments upon skin.'[47] The tests indicated that, since no powder blackening or tattooing had been found, the gun must have been fired from a distance of more than three inches from the victim's head, and from behind the ear at an angle which no-one intent on suicide would adopt.

Spilsbury's evidence effectively countered this case. After conducting tests with a similar pistol, he argued that there was little powder blackening even with the pistol held very close to the head. Any powder marks could easily have been removed by the escaping blood, or while the wound was being treated, without being noticed.[48] With a typical dramatic flourish Spilsbury produced a specimen of skin which had been shot at close range. One side of the wound showed powder blackening; the other had been wiped once, and all trace of powder blackening was gone. He also disputed that the angle of the wound was unusual, because

in a woman you often find very considerable range of movement of the shoulder joint owing to the habit of putting up the hair.[49]

Spilsbury, like the elder Glaister, always projected total confidence when in the witness box. Littlejohn, unfortunately, was faced with having to deny his own original report, and was completely flustered when Aitchison confronted him with a passage from a textbook by Sydney Smith, endorsed in a preface by Littlejohn himself, which implied that powder blackening from small arms was not always detectable. The wily Aitchison, however, omitted

Smith's further comment that such cases should always be decided by experiment with the weapon in question.[50]

Glaister followed Littlejohn into the witness box, but was unable to save the case for the prosecution. Although he now described the experiments on the leg, the prosecution's original decision not to make too much of this proved a mistake. Glaister, too, had a specimen of skin, which even after soaking in water for several months, clearly showed the marks of powder blackening from a shot at close range from Merrett's gun. This, however, had not been offered as a production, and Aitchison was able to ask why, if it had any importance, it was not put before the court earlier?[51] Although Glaister expressed perfect confidence that the blackening could not have been easily removed, he did not correct the poor impression made by Littlejohn.

In the end, there was a direct conflict of opinion between Spilsbury and the Scottish pathologists on the inferences to be drawn from the angle of the wound and the absence of powder marks. Smith, whose autobiography betrays strong dislike of Spilsbury, later exaggerated the 'worthlessness' of Spilsbury's own tests, which, he said, were conducted in London with a different gun and a different type of ammunition from that used in the crime.[52] This was unfair to Spilsbury, who also came to Edinburgh and, in Littlejohn's presence, performed tests on cardboard with Merrett's gun and the appropriate ammunition.[53] If Spilsbury was obstinate, it was in refusing to admit that the 'smokeless' cartridges he had used in London made less indelible marks on the skin than the Edinburgh ammunition. All the other experts claimed that the effects of the bullet used on Mrs Merrett would have produced indelible marks at a range of less than three inches. Aitchison, however, played effectively on popular feeling in his summing up: who could disbelieve Spilsbury, the man who had hung Crippen?

> I need not remind you that in this case we have had the great and learned assistance of Sir Bernard Spilsbury. I do not dispute that Professor Littlejohn and Professor Glaister are men of eminence, but I do not hesitate to say that there is no name in Britain, there is no name in Europe, on medico-legal questions, on the same plane as the name of Sir Bernard Spilsbury.[54]

The jury found the murder charge against Merrett not proven, and he served twelve months in jail for embezzlement. Time, of course, has judged in favour of Glaister and Smith. The astute William Roughead, editing the trial for the *Notable British Trials* series, expressed considerable doubt about the verdict, and 30 years later Merrett, then calling himself Ronald Chesney, justified these suspicions by committing suicide after murdering his wife and mother-in-law.

The elder Glaister, in his seventieth year at the time of the Merrett case, did not live to see his opinions vindicated. An earlier trial must also have been on his mind. In 1928 Roughead wrote to Glaister, asking him to check the record of his evidence in Merrett's trial before it was published in *Notable British Trials*. He added, with the audacity of long acquaintance: 'I see that our mutual friend Slater—about whom I had some correspondence with you in 1909—is again to the fore.'[55] Oscar Slater, finally released, was struggling to clear his name. Roughead, who edited both the Slater and Merrett trials for publication, was a shrewd observer, strongly hinting at Slater's innocence and Merrett's guilt. The ironies of history seemed to be moving against Professor Glaister at the end of his career.

The Merrett trial had all the ingredients to arouse public interest. The younger Glaister and Sir Sydney Smith both made great play of it in their respective autobiographies, although neither was called as a witness. Nevertheless, the trial seems to be almost the last example of an older period in forensic medicine. Aitchison made much of personalities, pitting Spilsbury's reputation directly against that of the Scottish pathologists. This type of personal confrontation was relished by the older generation of forensic pathologists, but developments in forensic science were making such courtroom battles obsolete. In Glasgow, as in London, forensic science was increasingly a matter of teamwork. Personalities might still seem larger than life, but they needed sober backing from the scientific laboratories.

Another aspect of the Merrett case is worth considering. Professor Glaister earned, for more than a week's work, the sum of just over £23, which had to cover his travel to Edinburgh (four days at 12s.6d. a journey) and other expenses.[56] He charged three guineas a day for attendance at the trial and his tests with Littlejohn in Edinburgh. Presumably he had to pay his son's expenses out of this, since the younger Glaister was not officially summoned. Although fees for court attendance and post-mortems had risen by a third since the Edwardian period, the cost of living had doubled. The costs of laboratory work were included in the standard charges of two guineas for four hours' work, although new methods such as the precipitin test were expensive to conduct. The elder Glaister, comfortably established and with his family off his hands, had little cause for concern; but those, like his son, who hoped to make a living from forensic medicine during the inter-war period, would find it a much less secure profession. Spilsbury was said to earn as little as ten guineas for a complicated case,[57] and, with less university backing than Glaister, began to overwork himself seriously to earn fees from coroners' inquests in order to maintain his standard of living.

'Young John', however, departed for a well-paid chair in Cairo, where the murder rate made Glasgow seem a sedate backwater. The Egyptian government provided ample resources for forensic medicine in the university, and it became something of an international showpiece. In Glasgow, the elder Glaister, never fearful of charges of nepotism, took one of his sons-in-law, Frank Martin, to assist him in his son's place. In the courtroom, Glaister's frail figure was now contrasted with the portly frame of Sydney Smith, who came over regularly from Edinburgh to appear for the defence. Relations were sufficiently amicable, however, for Smith to collaborate with the younger Glaister in publishing *Recent Advances in Forensic Medicine* (1931), in which Smith wrote about ballistics and Glaister about blood and hair.

Professor Smith and Professor Glaister continued the nineteenth-century tradition of vigorously contradicting each other's evidence. In the case of Robert Willox, disputes over the medical evidence led the defence to appeal against the verdict. In 1929 Willox, a man of 20, was tried for the murder of his elderly father, who was found battered to death in their flat. As with the other murdered parents in this chapter, the motive appeared to be financial gain; Willox, too, was forging his father's signature on cheques. With the aid of the kitchen door and a roll of linoleum which were brought into court, Glaister argued that the pattern of bloodstains showed that the victim had been attacked in the lobby of his flat, staggered into the kitchen and fallen on the floor, where he was beaten to death. Glaister found a few tiny stains of human blood on one of Robert Willox's jackets. A coal hammer in the flat was very clean—possibly it had been washed and dried—but traces of human blood were found between the hammer head and the shaft. Robert Willox's story was that he made tea for his father as usual, and that the old man ate a plate of vegetable soup. Willox then went out to play a game of billiards, which he won, and, when he returned, fainted on finding his father's battered body. This fall on the bloodstained floor accounted for the slight bloodstaining on Willox's clothes. Part of the prosecution's case was that the dead man had never eaten his meal, as unused dishes on the table showed, and that the son killed him before leaving to establish an alibi in the billiard hall. Glaister's post-mortem examination found no vestige of food in the stomach of the dead man. Glaister also tested the defendant's sanity, and found him fit to stand trial: it was not regarded as improper that the doctor who provided much of the prosecution's case should also deal with the prisoner in this manner.

Smith's testimony for the defence did not merely offer an alternative explanation of the physical evidence, but rather mischievously implied that the tests done by Glaister and Anderson were inadequate. Glaister had, as usual, carried out the precipitin test on the clothes of the accused, but did not attempt to find out whether the blood type was that of the murdered man. The defence implied, through Smith, that this could and should have been done.[58] Glaister's response, accepted by the judge, was that although blood typing was a routine process in hospitals for purposes of transfusion, it was not sufficiently accurate on bloodstains to be used in courts of law. In fact, the Home Office had been investigating the possible use of blood typing for forensic use since 1923, but there was difficulty in typing bloodstains more than 48 hours old.[59] Blood grouping had been offered as evidence on a few occasions in England, but not in a Scottish court. Although Glaister was, for legal purposes, in the right, his hostile reaction to questions about blood grouping seemed old-fashioned, and the defence tried to exploit this. Smith also made difficulties about Glaister's use of the precipitin test, arguing that he had not used a sufficient number of anti-sera to prevent a mistake.[60] This suggestion appears to have upset the normally imperturbable Glaister:

> We have gone over this test for two years in my laboratory and I do not give way to anybody regarding my knowledge of this test, and I have published a good deal about this test, and I do not want to have a red herring trailed over every substance.[61]

Smith, however, not to be outdone by Glaister in showmanship, was anxious to present his own information on blood testing as more up-to-date. A new technique was available to him in the benzidine test: if a small portion of a bloodstain were placed on filter paper with a mixture of benzidine and hydrogen peroxide, it produced a blue colour. This, although not a conclusive test for human blood, saved much time by eliminating stains of similar appearance such as rust or grease.[62] At first it was thought desirable to make a solution from the stain before testing, but the technique rapidly developed towards the modern system of allowing the searcher to dab a suspect stain with a prepared paper for an instant result. Further tests would then be made to check that the blood was human. Glaister was presented with Robert Willox's jacket and asked about the benzidene test:

[Q] ...Is there any simple and certain way of ascertaining at once whether blood is, or is not present in a given stain?
[A] No, not in fabric.
[Q] The benzedene [sic] test?
[A] That has to be applied with the material in solution. It is not done on the cloth. I wish it could be. It would be much simpler for me. [63]

Smith, on being asked the same question, produced his equipment and obligingly performed the benzidine test in court, directly from the fabric of the coat, to demonstrate that other untested stains were not blood.[64] Smith also contradicted Glaister's evidence on the time of death, arguing that a light meal of soup could well have been digested in the few hours which had passed before the body was discovered, and conversely, that if Robert Willox had committed the murder at the time alleged, rigor mortis should have been present by the time the body was found. When pressed, both he and Glaister admitted that there was considerable leeway for error in deciding the time of death.

In spite of the medical dispute over the bloodstains and the time of death, Willox was found guilty, since there was further evidence from neighbours that father and son had been heard quarrelling, and a motive was established. The judge, presented with the conflicting medical evidence, summed up thus:

where you are dealing with expert evidence you are in the region where there is room for controversy and difference of opinion, and juries naturally, and judges too, incline to a view that is favoured by the real evidence in the case, without necessarily attaching too much weight to the theories or speculations of the experts.[65]

When full transcripts are available, as they are of the Willox trial, it is tempting for the reader to put himself in the position of a juryman and come to his own conclusions on the basis of the evidence offered. This is largely a pointless task, especially over the medical evidence, since the historian cannot look over the shoulder of Glaister or Smith to see if they conducted their tests with complete propriety. Since the precipitin tests were complicated, and errors were possible, the best line for the defence was to attack the medical witnesses' competence. Both Smith and Glaister (in spite of their protestations), liked to 'win' a case, and battles of this kind were the result.

When the case went to appeal, the contradictions in the medical evidence were raised again, but the judges found that the weight of probabilities was with Glaister's version. Lord Clyde, the Lord Justice-General, used a phrase much relished by the younger Glaister: 'The line between suspicion and fact might be as slender as a hair, but it was as deep as the grave.'[66] He added that the jury would have been entirely justified in a verdict which went either way. Willox did not get the benefit of the doubt, but he was reprieved and sentenced to life imprisonment.

In a further murder case in 1931, Smith again contradicted Glaister's evidence on bloodstains. Glaister had tested for blood on the shoes of the accused, and found them heavily stained: Smith, who had not conducted any tests himself, argued that it was well known that leather tended to invalidate the precipitin test. The murder charge was found not proven, since there was little other evidence against the accused. It appears from Glaister's correspondence after the case, that he was much angered by Smith's assaults on his competence. The procurator fiscal took the unusual step after the trial had ended, of arranging a further test on the boots by another independent expert, who also detected the presence of blood.[67]

Glaister, however, was at last yielding to physical infirmity, and indicated to the university that he wished to retire. He continued to appear in the High Court until a few months before his death in December 1932, when he was in his 77th year. His age preoccupied counsels when they formally asked for his qualifications before questioning him, a fact which amused and flattered him. The following exchange arose over the death of Mrs Arbuckle, who the defence claimed, had died of natural causes. Counsel asked Glaister the victim's age.

[A] Between 65 and 70 was her age, I think.
[Q] That time of life is pretty old, is it not?
[A] In these days it is not as old as it used to be.[68]

Glaister was 72 at the time.

He vacated his chair in October 1931, but in 1932 he was asked to give expert advice in the last of his famous cases, particularly satisfying to him, perhaps, because both Spilsbury and Smith appeared for the defence.

The crime reporters who packed into the courtroom regarded these trials as straight fights between Smith and Glaister, or even between Edinburgh and Glasgow. Although the medical witnesses saw themselves as impartial, their audience was in no doubt that they had 'won' or 'lost.' Such was the popular view of the trial of Peter Queen, accused of strangling Chrissy Gall, the woman he lived with. After Queen came voluntarily to the police and made an incoherent statement, Chrissy Gall was found lying decorously and tidily in bed, her mob-cap and dentures undisturbed. Her neck was encircled by a piece of rope from the clothes pulley, with a half-knot to the right of her Adam's apple. There were no signs of struggle. Neighbours testified to the

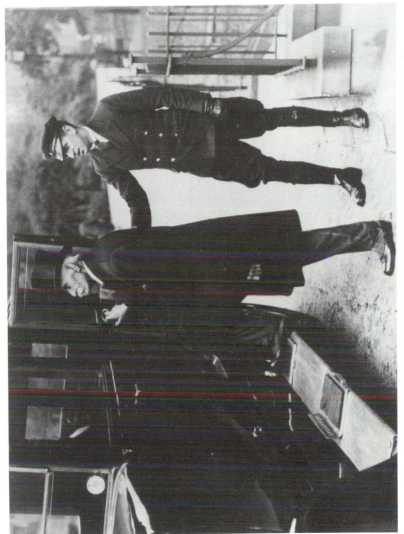

11a John Glaister Sr at the end of his career, departing for the High Court in full formal attire (GP)

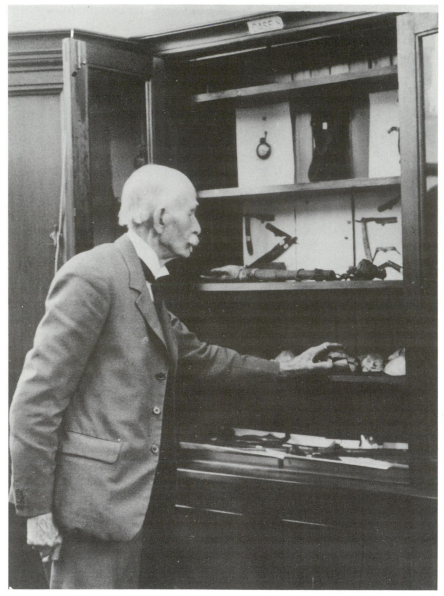

11b   John Glaister Sr with part of his 'Black Museum' (GP)

good relations between the young couple, and to Queen's patient temperament, though Chrissy Gall was depressed and addicted to drink. The defence, therefore, was suicide, although strangling with a ligature is a very uncommon method for suicides to adopt.[69]

Both sides were anxious to explain the placid appearance of the body: the defence claimed that this indicated suicide rather than murder, the prosecution that the victim had been too drunk to resist. Glaister, who was ill at the time of the arrest, did not conduct the post-mortem, and the doctors involved made no effort to analyse the stomach contents for the alcohol which was so important to the prosecution's case. Glaister, aged 76, was called to give an expert opinion on how the death could have occurred; he gave an athletic performance to demonstrate strangling positions, and was in the witness box for nearly five hours.[70] In his opinion, a fracture in the cricoid cartilage of the neck, just under the ligature, showed that more force had been used than a suicide could have mustered. Spilsbury stated, with his usual authority, that he had seen several cases of suicidal strangling, and that the loose knot and the position of the cord were consistent with such an explanation. Smith, more cautious, argued mainly on the relative absence of force—there was no bruising in the deeper tissues of the neck—and on the placidity of the body, though he knew this might be caused by drunkenness.[71] Both sides accepted that the medical evidence rested on the balance of probabilities, and the jury found Queen guilty, though they recommended mercy and he was reprieved. Smith, who did not share Spilsbury's total confidence in the suicide theory, had hoped for a verdict of not proven, and noted ruefully that 'in the only case where Spilsbury and I were in pretty complete agreement, the jury believed neither of us.'[72]

The press greeted the announcement of Glaister's retirement with fulsome columns appropriate to the man who had provided them with so much excellent copy. The *Evening News* published four interviews with Glaister, and expressed the opinion which, after three decades of enthusiastic press reports, was probably shared by most of Glasgow's newspaper-reading public:

> Many a time I have sat in a tense court-room watching the professor give evidence. Were I a criminal I would have been fascinated and yet frightened by the intensity of his gaze and the precision of his statements. He is exact to a second or a millimetre. His hand, as he speaks, grasps the rail of the witness box in seeming tension, for the knuckles are white and occasionally one can detect the faint blue ridge of a vein.
>
> He is the quintessence of justice. If there is anything that can be said in a man's favour he will say it. Yet his reports are never swayed by sugared sentiment. Some would say he is devoid of mercy, yet the sword of justice was never more evenly balanced than in his hands.[73]

CHAPTER FIVE

John Glaister II: An Uneasy Succession

John Glaister junior succeeded his father as regius professor in October of 1931, but, having to work out his notice in Cairo, he did not return to Glasgow until January 1932. The dynastic succession was bound to cause comment, and the new professor was aware that he would always be measured against his father. His credentials for the post were impeccable—nearly a decade of practical work with his father, his own intensive researches, three years of responsibility in an important overseas post, and a long list of scientific publications. He no longer submitted his father's name amongst his testimonials, as he could call upon some of the most distingished figures in British and European forensic medicine. Sir William Willcox, the senior pathologist at the Home Office, supported him; Uhlenhuth wrote warmly from Freiburg in praise of his work on blood and hair; Craigie Aitchison was prepared to vouch for his ability in the witness box.[1]

The Scottish press, obviously hoping for a new gladiator in the courts, greeted Glaister's appointment with much interest.[2] Some of Glasgow's senior pathologists were probably less welcoming, for Glaister was still only 40, and men like Andrew Allison and John Anderson had been appearing in Glasgow courts for a considerable time. Nor did Glaister's personality disarm all hostility, for there was an abrasive side to his character. Like his father, he was a slight, dark-eyed man, though the difference between their ages was emphasised by the elder Glaister's Victorian appearance and his son's suavely oiled hair and neat moustache—very much a figure of the Chamberlain era. Superficially, the younger Glaister seemed also to have inherited his father's supreme self-confidence, but in fact his character was more complex and introspective. He professed a religious faith, but was not a strict churchgoer; the Victorian certainties of his father's generation were possibly shaken by the brutal experience of war. Many of his interests, particularly in literature and the theatre, suggest a romantic and sentimental temperament struggling against the harsh demands of his profession. This, and the need to match up to his father's reputation, made him determined to assert himself.

Glaister found his Egyptian experiences very stimulating. Backed by a modern laboratory and a number of well-trained assistants, he worked on a wide variety of medico-legal cases. The Glasgow department, though well-equipped by British standards, could not match the generous provisions of

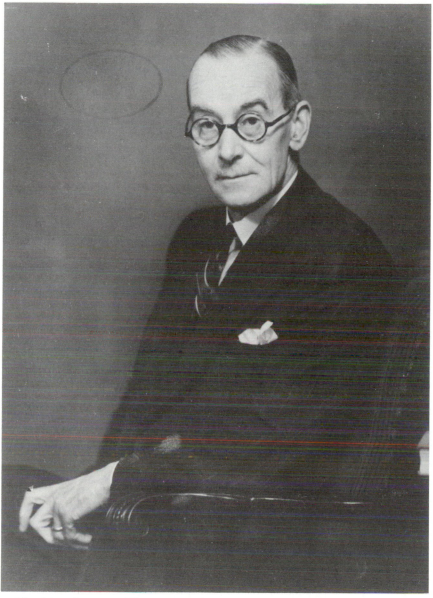

12   John Glaister Jr, fifth Regius Professor, at the time of his appointment (GP)

the Egyptian government, and, like Smith, Glaister came back to Scotland determined to improve the teaching and laboratory standards. The department's territory had shrunk, for the professor of public health had seized the opportunity of his father's retirement to take over the toxicological laboratory, and part of the museum on the upper floor had to be converted into a laboratory for forensic medicine.[3] The staff consisted of Glaister himself, with his brother-in-law Frank Martin as an assistant, and one technician.

About £1,500 was spent in providing the department with ultra-violet lamps, cine-cameras, and equipment for colour photography, all of which were commonplace in the teaching and court work of Cairo. Glaister was particularly intrigued by the possibilities of ultra-violet rays and x-rays in the detection of crime.[4] The beams of ultra-violet light, properly directed, produce fluorescence in many organic substances, and there was much work to be done in exploring this technique for medico-legal purposes. Ultra-violet light was particularly useful in identifying paper and other fibres; it could detect obliterated or altered handwriting, and might also be used to distinguish between the crystals of various types of drugs. Frank Martin began intensive work on it.[5] Like his father, Glaister was greatly interested in photography, and wished to give his students strong visual impressions; he also believed that colour photographs would convey more accurately to juries what the forensic investigations had uncovered.[6] (This intention was often foiled by prosecuting counsel, who considered it counter-productive to upset the stomachs of the jury with colour photographs).

Like many British medico-legists, Glaister hankered after the centralised forensic services found in Egypt and several European countries, and he planned to achieve more co-ordinated services in Glasgow.[7] He assumed that he would take over his father's work as expert witness for the Crown,[8] and that his department would occupy a key position if the forensic services in the West of Scotland were centralised. Instead, Glaister soon found himself virtually forced out of court work in Glasgow. There were two separate reasons for the failure of his hopes—the breakdown of his personal relations with the procurator fiscal, and the growth of an independent forensic service within the Glasgow police.

Glaister's ambitious plans were bound to upset established interests in Glasgow. In his autobiography, he argued that the 'old guard' were reluctant to consider any changes:[9] the senior pathologists, firmly based in the prestigious Glasgow hospitals, no doubt saw him as an interloper. Nevertheless, Glaister began to appear in court soon after his return, acting as second doctor to John Anderson. A particularly heavy diet of serious cases faced them in the Glasgow High Court in April 1932.

As head of the pathological laboratory at the Victoria Infirmary since 1913, and examiner for the Crown, John Anderson probably performed more post-mortems in his medical career than any other doctor in Scotland. He had worked as second doctor to the elder Glaister since 1913, but by the late 1920s was principal medical witness in many cases: when Glaister retired Anderson assumed the unofficial position of chief medical expert for the Crown. 'His appearance, voice, and manner could not be said to be impressive,' noted the *Glasgow Medical Journal* rather frankly, when Anderson died in 1939,[10] but his painstaking methods were valued by the fiscal, and the *Lancet* gave him credit, along with the elder Glaister, for maintaining 'the high plane on which the criminal administration in Scotland, and particularly in the West of Scotland, deservedly stands.'[11] A quiet man, who made no attempt to share the elder Glaister's limelight, Anderson's main research interest was not in criminal work, but in deaths under anaesthetic during surgical operations.[12]

The new Professor Glaister made an effective contribution in the trial of George Dollin, accused of murdering Mrs Mary Aitken by beating her to death. The circumstances of this case, sordid by any standards, were not merely a test of the pathologists' skills, but exposed in the harshest light the conditions of slum dwellers in the crowded tenements south of the river. The Aitkens and their five children shared a three-roomed tenement flat in Kingston Street with Dollin, the legal tenant: he invited the Aitkens to move in with him, since Aitken was unemployed and unable to get a house of his own. The prosecution alleged that, as part of the rent, Dollin enjoyed the favours of Mrs Aitken; apparently with the compliance of her husband, who spent much of his time lying in bed in a drunken stupor. Frequent drunken quarrels between Dollin and Mary Aitken caused the Aitkens to move out and lodge with a relative, but Mary Aitken left a number of items in the tenement, including a clinic card for one of her children. In spite of her home life, Mrs Aitken was a devoted mother, and was anxious about the card. Dollin told her that she must come and get the card personally; she agreed to meet him; they drank together and returned to the flat. In the close confines of the tenement buildings, the occupants could only retain their sense of personal respectability by 'keeping themselves to themselves', as several of the neighbours testified. Therefore, when sounds of violence came from the flat, as they did every weekend, nobody took any notice. Some time later, Dollin went to the police and claimed that Mary Aitken had died by falling against a table after drinking 'Red Biddy'—a mixture of cheap wine and methylated spirit.[13] After the post-mortem, a further defence that Mrs Aitken had died of a heart attack, was submitted.

John Anderson described the marks of violence on Mary Aitken's face and neck, and attributed her death to shock as a result of her injuries. Although the mitral valve of the heart showed signs of previous disease, Anderston thought it had compensated for this and was not the cause of death.[14] Glaister backed this up at some length, citing his five years' experience with the Ministry of Pensions, where he had investigated the heart problems of disabled ex-servicemen.[15] Sydney Smith, for the defence, argued that all the injuries could have occurred in a fall. Although he had not seen the body, he asserted that the heart condition, as described, might have caused death if the woman had been drunk and excited.[16] The prosecution made much of the tentative nature of his statements, and of the greater clinical experience of their own medical witnesses.

The judge urged the jury not to be unduly shocked by the habits of the lower classes: it was necessary, he said, to decide whether death had resulted from a premeditated attack or merely 'one of the ordinary scrambles which had taken place in a drunken bout from week-end to week-end.'[17] Dollin was convicted of murder by a majority verdict, and was reprieved at the last moment to serve a life sentence.

Although Glaister proved his usefulness to the prosecution in this and several other cases at the time, he then had a serious difference of opinion with the procurator fiscal. The cause of strife was Glaister's appearance for the defence in certain cases, to which the fiscal took exception, although Glaister had broken no formal rules.[18] The unwritten etiquette of Scottish forensic medicine discouraged the Crown's medical experts from appearing for the defence, though, as Sydney Smith's regular defence work in Glasgow makes clear, they were often prepared to appear for the defence outside their own territory. Glaister refused to accept the fiscal's views, and was then dropped from court work in Glasgow. Glaister did not name his adversary, but the fiscal for the Lower Ward of Lanarkshire at that time was J Drummond Strathern, who had occupied the position since 1918. His death, in the latter part of 1937, also marked Glaister's return to the High Court.

The incident is a mysterious one, since there is only Glaister's guarded account of it, and it is possible that Glaister's sense of his own importance made the situation worse. Medical ethics dictate that the doctor shall be a free agent, not bound to serve one side in a court of law; and the Scottish system also allows the medical experts to be precognosed, or examined, by the defence as well as the prosecution before a trial takes place. In the precognitions, as in court, it would be proper for the doctor to suggest that there is more than one way of interpreting physical signs. There is a standing temptation, however, for the medical expert who appears regularly for the Crown to be regarded as the prosecution's man, and the elder Glaister was often seen in this light. The son's more independent stance might therefore have seemed particularly irritating to a fiscal used to his father's ways. The younger Glaister took the chance to clarify his views when he added a new passage to his father's textbook in the seventh edition of 1942:

> What attitude should a medical witness assume towards solicitors and counsel for the other side? This is a question which often puzzles young medical men, and the following advice may save them anxiety. If a medical witness assumes the attitude that his duty is to aid the ends of justice, his path becomes quite clear. Should therefore, the prosecution or the defence desire to precognose a medical witness ... he should have not the slightest hesitation in submitting both his findings in, and views on, the case at issue, just as he had done for the side who first requested his professional services. The same facilities should be at the command of either the prosecution or the defence...[19]

This loss of court work was a serious blow to Glaister, and threatened to break the link his father had forged between the university and the courts in Glasgow. For nearly six years, one of the most highly qualified men in forensic medicine was denied the practical application of his work, though Frank Martin still represented the department occasionally in court. It was John Anderson and Andrew Allison who who coped with the notorious gang fights of the 1930s, examining the wounds, usually from broken bottles or razors hidden in the peaks of cloth caps, on the victims of the Norman Conks, Billy Boys, Bedford Boys and Bridgegate Boys.[20]

At this most difficult time in Glaister's career, his father and mother died of influenza in December 1932, within a few hours of each other. Failing health in the year before his death had finally diminished the elder Glaister's immense energy and his participation in professional work. He had been the most important influence on his son's life.

Courts outside Glasgow called the new Professor Glaister whenever they required special expertise, as in the 'Aberdeen sack case' of 1934, which was tried in Edinburgh because popular feeling in Aberdeen was so inflamed. A sack containing the body of an eight-year-old girl, Helen Priestly, was found in the ground-floor passageway of the tenement where she lived. She had been mutilated to simulate rape, and then asphyxiated. Since an extensive search for her was in progress, it was plain that her body must have been in one of the eight flats in the tenement: the main problem for the police was proving which of the neighbours was implicated. The post-mortem established that the child had been killed just after her meal in the middle of the day, at a time when everyone in the tenement had a convincing alibi except for Mrs Jeannie Donald. She and her husband, who were on bad terms with the child's parents, were both arrested, although there was no substantial evidence against them. While they were in custody, a massive forensic inquiry took place to find some link between the sack and the Donalds' flat, though Alexander Donald had to be released as his alibi proved unshakeable. Elaborate investigations failed to prove who owned the sack, but inside it were a few handfulls of washed cinders and household fluff.

The prosecution searched desperately for evidence, and a large group of forensic experts was called in: Sydney Smith, the chief medical witness, examined the flat minutely for bloodstains: although some were found, they could not be positively identified as the child's blood. More substantially, Smith tested a washcloth in the flat for blood, and found an unusual strain of intestinal bacteria, similar to those in the child's body.[21] The household fluff in the sack contained about two hundred different types of hairs and fibres, including human and animal hair. Glaister, as an internationally recognised expert on this subject, examined around 60 of the human hairs, trying to link Helen Priestly's hair with hairs found in the flat, and Jeannie Donald's hair with hairs found in the sack.[22] Evidence from the child's hair was not conclusive—she might, in any case, have entered the neighbouring flat at any time—but Glaister felt more positive about Jeannie Donald's hair than was normally possible with this kind of comparison. Mrs Donald's hair was permed; it also had an unusual, bulging irregularity which enabled Glaister to say in court that her hairs showed a 'striking similarity' with the

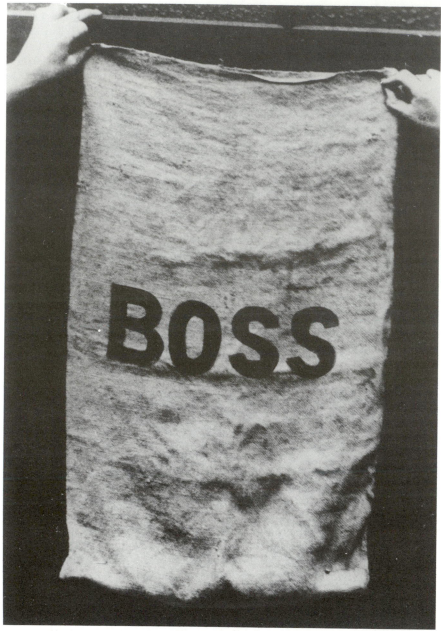

13   The sack in which Helen Priestly's body was found (Courtesy *Glasgow Herald* and *Evening Times*)

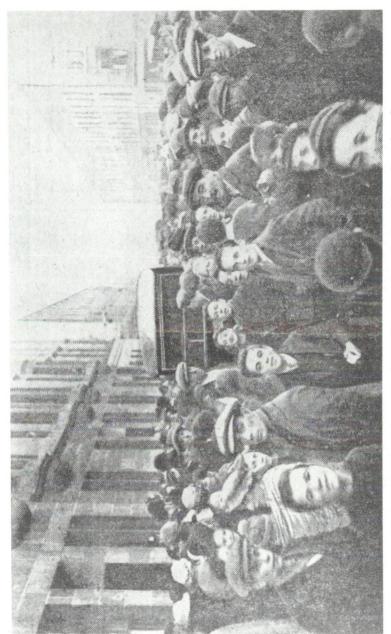

14 Aberdeen crowds surround the police van taking the Donaldsons from their flat (Courtesy *Glasgow Herald* and *Evening Times*)

hairs in the sack.[23] None of the individual links which the prosecution offered between Jeannie Donald and the sack were substantial in themselves, but the painstaking work of several doctors and scientists with hair, fibres, bacteria, cinders, and so on, collectively built up the case against her. For Mrs Donald the width of a hair might indeed have been as deep as the grave, for she was found guilty, though later sentenced to life imprisonment. Her motive was never made clear. Smith believed that she had merely slapped the child for being cheeky, the little girl had briefly lost consciousness, and Jeannie Donald, thinking she was dead, had simulated sexual assault to divert suspicion. When the child began to revive, Mrs Donald strangled her.[24]

Glaister appeared occasionally in other courts, including Ayr, Renfrew and Inverness, but the loss of Glasgow work affected his pocket as well as his prestige. At the end of the nineteenth century, when the university began to pay fixed salaries to its staff, many of the professors of clinical subjects were given relatively low salaries because they earned considerable fees from private practice. The elder Glaister's salary was fixed on this basis, because of his substantial outside income from court and other work. The younger Glaister's salary was similarly adjusted to take account of court fees; when court work in Glasgow was denied him, his income was not enough to support his standard of living, and was certainly far short of his generous salary in Cairo. He had fees from various other activities, such as checking death certificates for the crematorium, but nothing like the income, comparatively, of his father in the same post. In 1937 he had to write to the Principal in a way which he must have found humiliating:

> I believe that it is generally but wrongly assumed that the Crown work in Glasgow is, by rule, sent to the holder of this Chair; in fact, there is no obligation on the part of the local Procurator Fiscal to adopt this procedure since he is entitled to make his own selection. This work has been divided among several persons of whom I am not one...
>
> In effect, my position is that although I am remunerated on a part-time basis, I have been and am discharging the duties of a whole-time professor and my position differs from clinicians holding part-time Chairs since there is a wide public from which their private work is derived.[25]

The university Court agreed to pay Glaister a fixed salary of £1,100 a year for three years until the question of his other income was settled, but, fortunately for him, 1937 was his last year in the wilderness. From 1938 onwards, he was offered as much court work as he would accept.

The second reason why the forensic medicine department did not become part of a centralised forensic service at this time was the changing structure of the Glasgow police. At first this led to duplication of medico-legal work between police and university, but in the long run it led to the present division of functions between doctors and scientists.

As Norman Ambage has shown, the 1930s were a crucial time for the development of a forensic science service in Britain: under pressure from the Home Office, a Metropolitan Police laboratory was established at Hendon in 1934, and was soon followed by several provincial laboratories.[26] Whereas Hendon was directly administered by the police, the provincial laboratories were run by the scientists themselves. Both the younger Glaister and Smith were offered the directorship of Hendon, but turned it down because of the relatively low pay, limited research facilities, and lack of independence.[27] But in any case, the doctors could no longer undertake all manner of scientific tests, as they had in the nineteenth century. Even in the days of versatile medical experts like the elder Glaister, toxicological analysis was performed by chemists rather than doctors, although the doctors would still attempt chemical tests when necessary. Increasingly, however, they handed over the responsibility for analysis to chemists in the municipal service: most large cities in Britain had a public analyst (in Glasgow he was called the Corporation Chemist), who undertook both public health and police work. In the 1920s a medical man like Sydney Smith could still spend much time on ballistics, but as time went on, the scientists took over the matching of bullets to guns, and the doctors confined themselves to the effects of bullets on the human body.

Conversely, if a particular forensic technique was in constant demand by the police, it would be more useful and economical to develop routine procedures to be carried out by specially trained technicians rather than doctors or scientists. Fingerprinting was an early example of this: at first, doctors like the elder Glaister felt bound to master the technique, but it was taken over by specially trained policemen as its use became widespread amongst police forces. After 1945, the growth of road traffic accidents similarly encouraged the search for simpler methods of finding whether or not a driver was drunk.

Greater specialisation in the forensic services led inevitably to battles for control between doctors, scientists, and policemen. For once, the Glaisters, Smith and Spilsbury were in full accord, in that they all believed that the forensic services should be under the direction of medical men.[28] The doctors exerted a powerful fascination over the public, and were the best paid and most prestigious members of the forensic service. Many of them had the additional *cachet* of a university appointment. On the other hand, the kind of cases in which the doctors excelled represented only a small fraction of reported crime: the less sensational work of the chemist or the biologist had more to offer in solving everyday offences such as theft. The pathologists often dreamed of medico-legal institutes where they would have a commanding role: scientists and policemen were not always disposed to share this aim.

The Home Office initiative for a new scientific service in England and Wales was largely the work of a senior civil servant, Sir Arthur Dixon. The Scottish Office showed no such initiative, and the forensic services in Scotland were left to local discretion: before the 1930s, the Glasgow police had virtually no scientific services, and depended on Scotland Yard for help with fingerprinting and photography.[29] In December 1931, just before Glaister's return from

Cairo, Percy Sillitoe was appointed Chief Constable of Glasgow. Large, auto-cratic and very resourceful, Sillitoe immediately submitted plans to the Cor-poration for revitalising the force. As Chief Constable of Sheffield, Sillitoe, together with the police surgeon, had established a forensic science labora-tory, with a photographic laboratory and fingerprint section. The co-operative medical and scientific services were wide-ranging.[30] In Glasgow, Sillitoe rev-olutionised the police force, both in the organisation of manpower, and provision of forensic services. An efficient fingerprint laboratory was set up by Detective Sergeant Bertie Hammond, whom Sillitoe imported from Sheffield, and it also undertook work in photography and ballistics. The laboratory was under the direct control of the police, and its staff were police officers, though the Home Office disliked such arrangements, preferring scientists to be independent of police influence.[31]

More to Glaister's purposes, in 1933 Sillitoe persuaded the Corporation to provide a new mortuary. This building, at the foot of Saltmarket, was built, as Sillitoe reported, 'to hold a maximum of 24 bodies with equipment of the most modern and up-to-date type, with facilities for the scientific side of post-mortem examinations.'[32] At last the doctors could work in privacy and in reasonably hygienic conditions. Most of the makeshift mortuaries in the Glasgow area were demolished to make room for the garages of Sillitoe's new Flying Squad; while the mortuary of the Northern Division police station was turned over to the telephone switchboard. Although Sillitoe greatly improved the forensic services, they did not, considering the size of the city, match up to some of the new laboratories in the English provincial cities. Chief Constables, if left to themselves, naturally preferred to keep control over the forensic science service, and it was also cheaper, from the Corporation's point of view, to bring in outside experts when required than to maintain a large permanent staff. Since there was ample scientific expertise in the university and elsewhere in the city, there was less pressure for a large police service. Sillitoe, although interested in forensic medicine and science, was constrained financially: his great effort to provide the police with motor transport and better communications could be paid for only by cutting other police services.[33]

In 1931, Glasgow had eleven police districts, each with a police or 'casualty' surgeon. There was also the Physician to the Force, Robert Halliday, who acted as panel doctor to policemen requiring medical treatment. The police surgeons were all part-time—usually men in general practice. Under Sillitoe's new system, their numbers were reduced to seven (Frank Martin and Andrew Allison lost their posts), and the work of the Physician to the Force was redefined. Sillitoe wanted a full-time police physician to act as expert witness in the Sheriff and High Courts, and the new duties of the physician's office from 1932 included the requirement to carry out post-mortems and to exam-ine persons and articles for the fiscal, as well as working for the Glasgow police and other forces.[34] Halliday retired in 1935, and the police advertised for 'an expert on the medical aspects of crime.'[35] It proved difficult to find a man with the necessary expertise, and the post was not effectively filled until James Imrie was appointed in August 1936.[36]

In spite of Imrie's appointment, Glaister had no difficulty in returning to a prominent place in the Glasgow courts. In fact, there was work for several medical experts. Since there were fewer police surgeons, Imrie was much occupied with clinical work, and his duties still included medical treatment for policemen: the Glasgow police establishment, both in medicine and forensic science, was simply not large enough to cope with the medico-legal needs of the city. The fiscal still had to use independent experts such as John Anderson, who had a laboratory in the Victoria Infirmary, and Andrew Allison, whose private laboratory was in the basement of his house. Although Glaister was not on good terms with the fiscal, he avoided any break with the police, to whom he had given lectures on forensic medicine for several years before he left for Cairo. Glaister also established a cordial relationship with James Imrie.

Glaister did not simply slip back into court work when his battle with the fiscal ended. By 1938 he was as well known across the nation's breakfast tables as his father. When he was appointed to the regius chair, he had a solid scientific reputation, and his name, naturally, was familiar in Glasgow, but in 1936 he sprang to national prominence. The reason for this sudden fame was, of course, the celebrated Ruxton trial. That Glaister was called in as expert witness was, for him, entirely a matter of fortunate coincidence. If the murderer of Mrs Ruxton and Mary Rogerson had lived in Glasgow, the fiscal would never have summoned Glaister. As it happened, the murderer lived in Lancaster, but the fragments of the two dismembered bodies were found in a stream near Moffat, about 50 miles south of Glasgow. The local fiscal, needing a medical expert of uncommon skill, immediately looked towards Edinburgh. But Sydney Smith, then the most famous medical detective in Scotland, was, as it happened, in Australia, puzzling over a severed arm disgorged by a shark; when he got back to Scotland, he was summoned mainly to confirm findings already made. The fiscal called an Edinburgh pathologist, Gilbert Millar, and also the Professor of Anatomy at Edinburgh, James Couper Brash; but the case required an extraordinary amount of effort from a forensic team. And so it was Glaister who carried out a substantial part of the medico-legal work in the Ruxton case, and acted as chief medical witness to a court in Manchester.

A murder which particularly interests the forensic scientist is not necessarily fascinating to the general public, and *vice versa*. If a murder passes into the national mythology, the human circumstances are usually more memorable than the medical or scientific evidence. George Orwell gave some thought to this subject a few years after the Ruxton case, in an essay entitled *Decline of the English Murder*:

> ...one can construct what would be, from a *News of the World* reader's point of view, the 'perfect' murder. The murderer should be a little man of the professional class—a dentist or a solicitor, say—living an intensely respectable life somewhere

in the suburbs, and preferably in a semi-detached house, which will allow the neighbours to hear suspicious sounds through the wall. He should be either chairman of the local Conservative Party branch, or a leading Nonconformist and strong Temperance advocate. He should go astray through cherishing a guilty passion for his secretary... Having decided on murder, he should plan it with the utmost cunning, and only slip up over some tiny, unforeseeable detail. The means chosen should, of course, be poison.[37]

If we put aside consideration of the Ruxton case as a personal tragedy and see it in Orwell's terms as a macabre public entertainment, then it falls somewhat short of his Crippenesque ideal in its details, but is close to it in spirit. Buck Ruxton was a doctor, living in a terraced house in Lancaster, and very sensitive about his social status; Mrs Ruxton knew that she could rouse him to fury by calling him 'low born'.[38] He was not as respectable as he seemed to his patients, for he was not married to Mrs Isabella Ruxton, the mother of his three children, who had changed her name to his by deed poll. Nor was Ruxton his original name, since he was an Indian, and he too had used the deed poll to acquire the rather odd anglicised version. The supposed guilty relationship was not his, but Mrs Ruxton's, whom he continually suspected of affairs with other men, but his passionate jealousy was a classic motive for murder. He probably did not plan to murder his wife, but when she returned home late one night from what he imagined was an assignation, he strangled her while their children slept upstairs. There was the additional horror of the death of Mary Rogerson, the Ruxtons' twenty-year-old nursery-maid, killed because she witnessed her mistress's death. At that point, however, Ruxton attempted to disguise his crime with the requisite amount of misdirected cunning, and the forensic evidence was crucial both in identifying the bodies and bringing evidence against the murderer. This forensic evidence was so varied and impressive that it appealed equally to the public and to the specialists.

The Ruxton case features in detail in two autobiographies,[39] and is also the subject of an entire technical work, *Medico-legal Aspects of the Ruxton Case*, which Glaister wrote with Brash. A reader of the autobiographies of Glaister and Sydney Smith will receive the strong impression that each writer solved the case almost single-handed, and indeed, the two experts virtually ignored each other's existence in their autobiographies, even though they confronted, or assisted, each other for several decades.[40] In Scottish courts, a medical witness is not permitted to hear the evidence given by other medical men, and the memoirs were possibly written on the same principle. A third account, in Douglas Grant's history of the Glasgow police, redresses the balance by ignoring the doctors and concentrating on the fingerprint work done by the police laboratory.[41] In fact, the most important aspect of the Ruxton case, as the more technical study shows, was the highly sophisticated degree of medical and scientific teamwork, typical of modern forensic inquiries into serious crimes. Smith and Glaister liked to cast themselves in the role of the old-fashioned medical detectives when they wrote of their famous cases, but the real heroism in the Ruxton case was not that of any single individual, but of

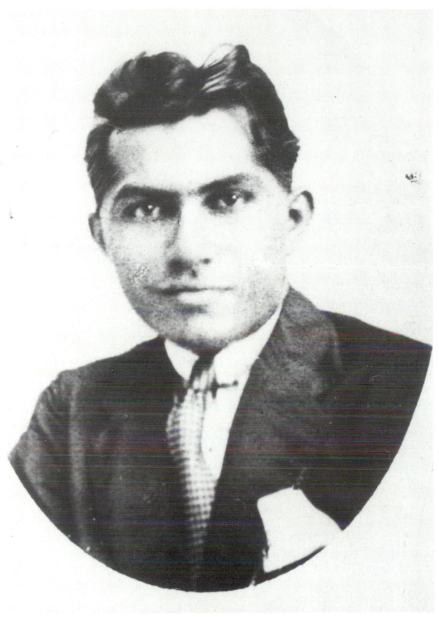

15   Dr Buck Ruxton (GP)

several men applying themselves to laborious and gruesome tasks. Apart from Glaister, Smith, Brash and their assistants, there were two dental experts, radiographers, an entomologist (to help determine time of death by the age of insect larvae on the bodies), and the photographic and fingerprinting expertise of the Edinburgh and Glasgow police.

Ruxton was determined that the bodies should not be identified, and must have spent the whole night after the murder draining them of blood in the bath and dismembering them. He not only cut each body into several pieces, but removed internal organs and much of the flesh, together with anything which could assist identity, such as eyes, prominent teeth, and birthmarks. He parcelled up the remains in several bundles, wrapped in newspaper and pieces of sheeting, and left them in the locked bathroom while he dealt with visitors and took his children to a friend's house. He then drove to Moffat, where he threw several of the parcels into the stream and others into ditches and other places. A tourist discovered some of the remains about ten days later, by which time the stream had been in spate and carried away many of the parts. Some were found later, scattered over a wide area, but much was still missing, including one of the torsos. So gross was the disfigurement, that Glaister and the other doctors believed at first that the bodies were a man and a woman. But in spite of this immense effort to conceal identity, Ruxton committed the necessary mistake. He wrapped the fragments in pieces of bedlinen, a blouse, a pair of child's rompers, and sheets of newspaper. The newspaper not only provided a guide to the possible date of the murder, but was a local edition limited to the Morecambe area, and so fixed a geographical area as well. Since the bodies had been cleanly divided with a knife, and the teeth removed neatly with an appropriate tool, the medical men immediately suspected that the murderer had some anatomical knowledge.

The remains were removed to the University of Edinburgh, and labelled 'Body no. 1' (Mary Rogerson) and 'Body no. 2' (Mrs Ruxton). The immediate task was to reconstitute them. Professor Brash worked on this grisly anatomical jigsaw, but fitting the parts to the right body was no easy task, since so many of the pieces were still missing. With careful articulation of bones, recorded at all points with x-ray photographs, Brash produced a satisfactory reconstruction, and realised that the bodies were those of two women. One head was of proportions within the range of statistical overlap between men and women, but was convincingly fitted to body no. 2, where the sex organs were intact. The other head had a small larynx which was obviously female, and also pieces of facial skin which showed no signs of a beard; this meant that body no. 1 could also be identified as a woman's, although the trunk was missing. Ruxton's action in draining the bodies of blood and removing viscera also retarded the normal processes of decay, and it was possible, after microscopic examination, to identify some of the pieces of flesh, which included *three* female breasts.

Fortunately for the investigation, the appearance of the bones allowed a more accurate identification than if the two women had been closer in age. At Mary Rogerson's age (20), sutures in the bones of the skull were not entirely closed; calicification of the ends of bones and teeth was not complete,

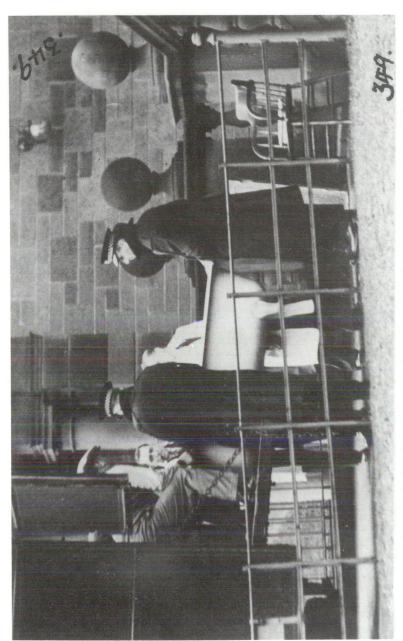

16   Ruxton's bath arriving at the forensic medicine department for examination (GP)

and the wisdom teeth had not erupted: this distinguished her from the more mature Mrs Ruxton (34). These decisions on the sex and age of the bodies, together with the newspaper wrappings, led the police investigation to Lancaster, where two women were reported missing. The press became increasingly excited with every police announcement, and as more remains were found. A workman by the side of the Glasgow-Carlisle road discovered a bundle of newspaper and joked to his mates, 'Be careful as we might find a piece of Mrs Ruxton.' The paper contained a foot.[42]

Meanwhile, Bertie Hammond at the Glasgow police laboratory followed his own line of inquiry. The hands of body no. 2 were missing, but it was possible, with immense care, to make a fingerprint and palm print from the wrinkled skin on the left hand of body no.1. These matched prints in Ruxton's house.[43] Later, the right hand of body no. 2 was found, and although the outer skin (epidermis) had been shed, many of the ridges were still visible on the underlying skin (dermis) of the thumb, and were photographed. This incomplete thumbprint had sixteen points of similarity with thumbprints in the Ruxton house: this was enough to satisfy Hammond, since eight similarities were regarded as statistically significant, but the dermal print was not used in court.[44] The clothing found with the bodies was clearly identified as Mary Rogerson's, and a further technical feat by a Manchester expert in the testing of textiles showed that unusual flaws in the selvedges of the sheeting found with the bodies matched bedlinen in Ruxton's house.

Glaister, with Millar and Frank Martin, examined the bodies carefully for identifying features, and to establish the cause of death. Body no. 2, in spite of severe mutilation, showed signs of asphyxiation, since the hyoid bone in the neck was broken, and small haemorrhages were apparent in the lungs. It was not possible to determine the cause of death in body no. 1. The medical team noted that areas of mutilation in both bodies coincided exactly with places where the women were known to have distinguishing features: skin had been stripped from an arm where Mary Rogerson had a large birthmark, flesh removed from the toe where Mrs Ruxton had a bunion, and so on. In fact, the areas of mutilation corresponded so closely with the women's distinctive features, that this actually increased the probability of their identity. Ruxton's attempt to disguise dental patterns was also foiled by the dental team, who could distinguish between the sockets of teeth which had been removed some time previously, and those removed by the murderer. Both women had teeth missing in the same places as the sockets of old extractions in the bodies. Glaister and Smith had, as it were, to re-enact the dismemberment and calculate how long it would take someone with medical knowledge to do it: they knew, by the draining of the blood, that the operation had been performed soon after death, and reckoned that five hours was the minimum time.[45] Given Ruxton's known movements, he must have done the work in his own house.

Glaister then visited the house in Lancaster and applied the benzidine test for the presence of blood. Consequently, a very large number of objects, including wallpaper, skirting boards, carpets and fittings, were transported back to the University of Glasgow in a large furniture van for further testing.

The entire contents of the bathroom, including parts of floors and walls, were taken to Glasgow, and the room reconstructed. Copious bloodstains were revealed, even though Ruxton had done some preliminary cleaning and then called in a charwoman to finish it. Ruxton had a badly cut hand—he may possibly have done it deliberately, or accidentally while dismembering the bodies—and claimed that this was the source of all the blood in the bathroom. Glaister traced the pattern of bloodstains and argued that this was an unlikely explanation. In particular, although Ruxton had cleaned the inside of the bath with care, blood had run over the rim and down the side panels.[46] It is noteworthy, however, that Glaister did not conduct tests to see if the blood-stains were of the same blood group as Ruxton's—this test was still con-troversial and difficult to perform on any but very fresh bloodstains.

This brief description hardly does justice to the forensic complexities of the Ruxton case, which, as has been mentioned, filled an entire book. A lesser combination of these discoveries, with the fingerprint evidence, would prob-ably have convicted Ruxton, but together they were unassailable by the defence. Defence counsel sought advice from Spilsbury and other leading experts, but were unable to do more than query minor points: no medical witness took the stand on Ruxton's behalf. To add an extra rococo flourish, there was Professor Brash's remarkable piece of anatomical camera work: he had superimposed a life-size studio photograph of Mrs Ruxton's head on to a photograph, aligned on the same plane, of the skull of Body no. 2. He had calculated the exact size of her head from a tiara she was wearing in the studio portrait, and the dimensions of the two photographs corresponded remarkably. Although this evidence was accepted in court, it could do no more than make the identification of the bodies slightly more probable, but Brash's virtuoso performance was greatly admired by the other medical experts.

Glaister was the first of the expert witnesses for the Crown, and stood in the witness box for the best part of two days. His presentation was extremely precise and clearly articulated, and he dealt with cross-examination as brusquely as his father;

> [Q] Of course, there may be many, many occasions when blood is spilled in a bathroom. For example, you could cut yourself shaving and there would be blood?
> [A] I should be amazed if I cut myself shaving and subsequently found on the side of the seat what I saw in this case. [47]

Glaister's manner of giving evidence differed from his father's in that he made no attempt to answer every question put to him, but referred counsel to the evidence of other expert witnesses. Questions on anatomy were Brash's territory, for example.[48] By 1936, no medical witness could assert all-round competence, especially over evidence as complicated as in the Ruxton trial: it was clear that the forensic sciences were reaching a degree of specialisation hardly possible even a decade previously.

The hanging of Buck Ruxton brought Glaister much public attention, and established him in the forefront of British forensic medicine. Forensic experts were used to having their work exaggerated by the press, but during the Ruxton case Glaister was credited with almost miraculous powers. The *Sunday Dispatch* claimed that he could tell the age, sex and weight of a body from a single hair.[49] He was invited to lecture to police forces all over the country, and the Ruxton trial provided him with the opportunity for a *bravura* lecture both to his own students and the Glasgow police, for many years. In 1938 he was able to resume work as expert witness for the Crown in Glasgow.

Some of those connected with the department in later years thought that the Ruxton business had been rather overdone, since its notoriety tended to overshadow less sensational but necessary routine work. Yet the Ruxton case deserves its central position. It increased both self-confidence and public respect in the fledgling forensic services of the 1930s. It finally signalled an end to the days of the medical detective investigating a complex crime almost single-handed. It also showed the high degree of co-operative teamwork which was possible between the police, the universities, and other outside experts, even though there was no central organisation. Since the various forensic services grew without any central planning, informal co-operation was essential to their success. Rightly or wrongly, this was to become the characteristic shape of the forensic services in Glasgow, and indeed, in Britain.

CHAPTER SIX

The Rise of Forensic Science 1939-1962

When Glaister returned to work for the fiscal in 1938, he soon had more than enough to do, and the outbreak of war increased the pressure even further. Like his father, Glaister seems not to have kept a log of his medico-legal cases, but there is other evidence to suggest what the weight was in these years.

Many forensic experts have, reasonably enough, seen their memoirs as a nest egg in their retirement. They naturally concentrate on their famous murder cases, and sometimes give the impression that these take up most of the medical detectives' time. In fact, since murders are few, most of the work concerns suicide, fatal accident or sudden death. Glaister expected that war would greatly increase the number of murders, with more guns in circulation and more men trained in unarmed combat. He was wrong: the annual numbers of murders and culpable homicides known to the police in Glasgow during the war was much the same as during the 1930s: an erratic figure, usually between ten and sixteen, about half of all homicides in Scotland. Guns were used more often, but premeditated use of a weapon was not common. It should be remembered that the homicide figures at this time included substantial numbers of infanticides and botched abortions. Of the 27 murders and 27 culpable homicides known to the Glasgow police in the five years 1935-39, eleven were of newborn children and seven of women dying as the result of an illegal abortion.[1]

Nevertheless, Glaister's work did increase in wartime. All the medical services were tightly stretched, and he was called to other parts of Scotland, and to assist with courts martial. The number of suicides in Glasgow fell during the war, to an average of about 65 a year, compared with an average of 95 in the five pre-war years; but this was more than compensated by fatal accidents (not counting traffic accidents), which suddenly rose from 215 in 1939 to 284 in 1940, and remained high for the rest of the war, the result of greater fire risk, and danger from bomb-damaged buildings.[2] The police surgeons and hospital pathologists dealt with most of the routine cases, but their own resources were under pressure.

Frank Martin's health was failing; he left the department in the early 1940s and died in 1943, and so Glaister had no full-time assistant, though James Imrie took over some of the teaching. Glaister also had a technician and a

93

trainee technician to help him in the laboratory. When two doctors were needed on a case, Glaister often worked with Frank Reynolds, the pathologist to Glasgow's municipal hospitals. Both the university laboratory and Glaister's house were damaged in bombing raids, making life even more difficult.

Police statistics show increased use of firearms in assaults and homicides during the war. The Glasgow police laboratory carried out ballistic tests in only two cases in 1942, rising to twenty in 1945. As a result of this and other wartime needs, the work of the Fingerprint Bureau was extended in the early 1940s, and it was rather cumbersomely renamed the Fingerprint, Photographic and Scientific Bureau. In 1945, all these activities became separate branches of the Identification Bureau, and the Scientific Branch steadily expanded until it became the largest forensic science laboratory in Scotland.[3] It started with lesser offences such as housebreaking, but was soon engaged in solving more serious crimes.

The police laboratory began to take over scientific tests previously the task of medical experts, but there was a period of overlap. Wartime needs encouraged interest in ballistics, but the laboratory also offered a wider range of chemical and microscopical tests for hairs, fibres, glass, metals, paints, paper, explosives, plastics, and many other substances, together with investigations of handwriting, typewriting, laundry marks, and so on. In England, the new Home Office laboratories of the 1930s had taken away much of this type of work from the medical experts: the process was slower in Scotland, partly because the courts had great respect for the doctors, who were seen as impartial witnesses. Unlike the Home Office laboratories in England, the Glasgow forensic laboratory was staffed by policemen, and was part of the police establishment. Some argued that this made it seem an arm of the prosecution rather than an independent scientific body.[4] Doctors had more prestige in court than policemen, and for a time the fiscals insisted on calling medical experts to back up the police evidence.

The scientific laboratory was originally staffed by two experienced policemen from the Fingerprint Bureau: Detective Lieutenant George Maclean, and Detective Constable George Sowter, both trained in ballistics. They were joined before the war by a police recruit with a degree in chemistry, James McLellan. McLellan, a future chief constable of Lanarkshire, specialised in infra-red photography of powder burns, and carried out chemical tests for nitrite on both victims and suspects. Nitrite is produced by combustion when a gun is fired, and was useful evidence if found on a suspect's hands. For some years, the scientific takeover proceeded slowly, with university experts being consulted in serious cases, as the following examples demonstrate.

In 1940, the wife of a soldier on leave was killed by a bullet which passed through her mouth and out of the back of her neck. The soldier's story was that during a quarrel his wife had pointed the rifle at him (possibly not realising it was loaded), and that it went off accidentally when he tried to take it from her. This was a Stirlingshire case, and the ballistic evidence came from Mr A E Martin, a Glasgow gunsmith, who matched the bullet to the gun. Glaister and Martin experimented with the gun, and estimated the probable distance of the shot at about 18 inches. From fragments of bullet in the wall and the pattern of bloodstains, they traced the path of the bullet, and reported that the rifle had been pointing horizontally or slightly downwards at approximately 4 feet 5 inches from the floor. They looked for powder blackening on the woman's bare arms to confirm her husband's story that she was clutching the gun, but found none. The prosecution therefore claimed that the woman could not have been holding the gun because it was too far away from her face when it went off, and at too high an angle. Sydney Smith, for the defence, argued that a horizontal shot might imply self-defence, and that the woman could have grasped the gun without receiving powder burns. Since there were no witnesses, nor any proof of motive on the husband's part, the forensic evidence was inconclusive, and the verdict was one of not proven.[5]

In this case it was the doctors and a gunsmith who gave evidence on firearms: Smith, in particular, was much interested in ballistics. Within a few years, however, the Glasgow police laboratory provided most of the evidence in firearms cases, but still deferred to the medical witnesses. In late 1945 and early 1946 several shootings took place, and by this time the procedure was well established. The police experts attended the post mortem, and took away evidence such as bullets and clothing. If they had a suspected weapon, they fired from it similar bullets to those used in the crime to see if the markings tallied: they also took photo-micrographs of bullets, to be used as evidence in court. The police noted the amount of pressure needed to pull the trigger, and estimated the distance of the shot, with particular attention to powder blackening on body or clothing. McLellan took infra-red photographs of clothing, and tested swabs from suspects' hands for nitrite. On several occasions, Glaister came to the fingerprint bureau to watch the police tests; he also read their reports and vouched for their accuracy. In some cases he carried out chemical tests himself to confirm the police findings. At this stage, the fiscal was effectively using Glaister to give a seal of approval to the police procedure, and also to back it up in court if necessary, since scientific experience might go for nothing if not ably presented in the witness box.

Glaister's courtroom technique appeared to advantage in a trial in 1946. In an apparently motiveless crime, a man was killed by a shot in the abdomen, after being approached by two brothers in the Dumbarton Road. The gun was dropped as they ran off; later, one of the brothers was arrested and charged with murder. The police team tested the weapon and the victim's clothing, but found no traces of nitrite on the accused. The defence claimed that the gun had gone off accidentally while the three men were examining it. Both Glaister and the police argued against the possibility of accident, because of freak markings on the victim's clothes. Glaister's report stated that:

a bullet had passed through the trousers, shirt and semmit [vest];

that it had been fired when the firearm was in contact with the clothing, and that the muzzle end of the weapon had been pressed so heavily against the clothing that the heat generated by the firing had produced a complete outline of the muzzle end of the weapon which could be clearly seen on the outer surface of the trousers and more faintly on the pocket of the trousers.[6]

Glaister, as skilled as his father in keeping the jury's attention, left the witness box to demonstrate how he thought the shot had been fired: he held the dead man's trousers against the defence counsel, Mr John Cameron KC, and thrust the pistol firmly into the belly of the future peer.[7] The verdict was culpable homicide, and the accused was gaoled for six years.

A few months later the police mounted an intensive search for the murderer of a retired policeman, James Straiton, killed while tackling a burglar at a neighbouring house. The neighbour, James Deakan, returned home with his wife from the cinema one night and saw a light in an upstairs window: suspecting that his house had been burgled, he went to ask the former policeman for help. The front door of Deakan's house was locked from inside, and as Deakan and Straiton were trying to get in at the back, two men came down the stairs brandishing guns; Straiton and his neighbour tackled them, and Straiton was shot dead. The burglars escaped, one in his stocking feet, for he had left his shoes in the garden when he climbed the drainpipe to get into the house. Within a few days, the police arrested John Caldwell, a twenty-year-old army deserter: he was trapped by a classic combination of ballistic techniques and methodical police procedure. In the police laboratory, George Maclean had recently examined a bullet fired to break the lock of a bedroom door in another case of housebreaking. He compared this with the bullet from Straiton's body, and found they were from the same Colt automatic pistol. After a third housebreaking, where the thief threatened the occupant with a gun, a partial fingerprint remained on a broken window pane. In all three houses the method of entry was by climbing the drainpipe and the police concentrated on tracing criminals known to use this method. The fingerprint led them to Caldwell. In his father's house was a watch stolen from the house where the gun that killed Straiton had been fired to break the lock. Glaister carried out the post-mortem on Straiton, and examined Caldwell for an injury said to be inflicted during the fight, but the police provided their own ballistic evidence without help from the medical experts.[8] The young man was hung for murder, and his accomplice sent to a mental institution.

Another case in which doctors and police worked closely together was the death of a four-year-old girl, Betty Alexander. She lived with her parents in Glasgow's cosmopolitan area of Garnethill, behind Sauchiehall Street. She was last seen playing with another child on the evening of 7 October 1952, and an intensive search began when she did not come home. Nevertheless, her body was not found until three days later, on the steps leading down into a small enclosed yard behind the Sick Children's Dispensary, 200 yards from her home. Her coat was folded neatly into a pillow under her head, and she had died after a brutal sexual attack. The yard was accessible only through a door from the dispensary, or through the locked door into the outside lane; but the police decided it was possible to climb the ten-foot wall carrying the child's body. Just before her death, she had eaten some soup, which was not accounted for at her home or elsewhere. She had obviously been dead for a considerable time before she was found, but neither the precise time nor place of death could be determined.

Glaister, Imrie, and Maclean were the focus of an intensive forensic inves-

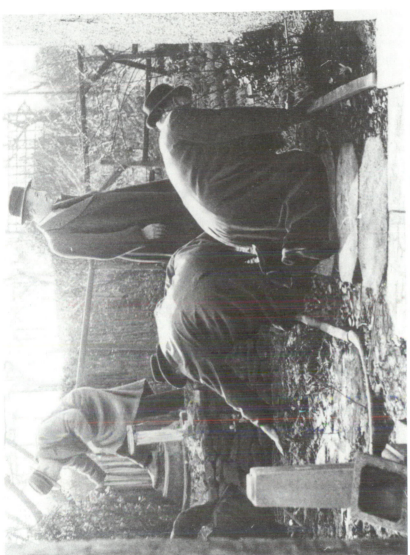

17   Detectives looking for clues in the Straiton murder case (Courtesy *Glasgow Herald* and *Evening Times*)

tigation, carried out at the scene of the crime and in the university laboratory. A nearby house and its occupants were subjected to minute scrutiny. The experts examined carpets, furniture, clothing, cat hairs, fingernail scrapings, and other items, but no conclusive evidence was found. The crime, the first of its kind in Glasgow for thirty years, caused great revulsion in the city, but no arrest was ever made. Glaister worked exclusively on the case, and was constantly on call in case the police required him. A case of this complexity pushed routine work into the background, and stretched the forensic services to the limit. But the key of interchange had been lost in spite of this enormous effort.

In the post-war years, Glaister's laboratory lacked the resources to cope with all the basic work in forensic science, and the police inevitably took over much of it. At this time, many forensic scientists were resentful that their own special knowledge was sometimes outweighed in court by the prestige of medical experts with limited scientific training—and the doctors were also more highly paid than the scientists. Sheer pressure of work and the demand for more specialised services loosened the medical grip. In 1965 the Glasgow police put their scientific laboratory on a new footing when they began to appoint highly qualified scientists who were not policemen, though still under the general direction of the Chief Constable. When Scottish local government was reorganised in 1975, the police became the responsibility of Strathclyde Regional Council, serving the whole of West Central Scotland. The Strathclyde Police Forensic Laboratory expanded to meet this need.

The responsibilities of doctors and scientists still overlapped, and the doctors still undertook a wide range of medical tasks. Glaister carried out clinical examinations, and had a particular interest in homosexual offences. He continued to take life insurance work, and to check death certificates for the crematorium. One sign of specialisation, however, was the department's reduced interest in whether an accused person was fit to plead. The elder Glaister regarded psychiatric examinations as a normal part of his duties, but in his son's time this task was largely left to doctors with special qualifications.

Glaister was well aware of the possible split between forensic medicine and forensic science, especially as his earlier hopes for a single Medico-legal Institute in Glasgow had been frustrated. He recorded the expansion of his subject in his own editions of his father's textbook, which he managed to revise six times between 1938 and 1962. He was also anxious to make the university a centre for research in forensic medicine and science.

Research was expanding during the 1930s, when a number of postgraduate students came to study with Glaister, either for a higher degree, or to extend their knowledge of forensic medicine. He gave informal instruction to students from several countries, and, fittingly enough, it was a student from Egypt who received the department's first Ph.D., for a study of the medico-legal application of the blood groups.[9] Post-graduate work tailed off after 1939, but Glaister believed that demand would rise again after the war, as he explained in a letter to the Principal in August 1944.[10] His undergraduate lecture classes were large in the 1930s, with about 90 lawyers and 170 medical students: these numbers, too, would expand after the war as soldiers who had postponed their studies returned.

Glaister reminded the Principal that the salary of the regius chair was still part-time, and that the professor needed to support himself with outside fees. Given the pressure of criminal work, there was a danger that the department's research and teaching would be submerged by routine investigations. Glaister proposed that after the war he should be placed on a full-time salary; in return, he would give up all but a small number of his outside cases, and concentrate on his university duties, even though this might mean a reduction in his income. In particular, he hoped for a postgraduate training course, the first of its kind in Britain, drawing on the expertise of the police, the courts, and the City Analyst's department. This suggestion probably reflected Glaister's own preferences: he enjoyed the excitement of an interesting murder case, but had little liking for routine pathology; indeed, he always seemed happier behind a microscope than in the mortuary. In the event, the University offered him an improved salary of £1,200, still assuming some supplementation from private fees. The Finance Committee noted ominously, however, that the full-time chair was personal to Glaister, and when he retired it might well be commuted to a lectureship—the same recommendation that had been made on his father's appointment nearly sixty years previously.[11] For quite other reasons, trying to consolidate forensic medicine in the universities at this time was to swim against the stream.

Glaister had overestimated the possible increase of crime during the war, but he predicted correctly that demand for forensic services would rise after the war. Not only did violent crimes increase, but the rapid advance of forensic science allowed it to offer a much wider range of services in criminal investigation.[12] The British universities seemed better placed to meet increasing demand than at any previous time. From 1933, forensic medicine was a compulsory subject in the curriculum of English medical schools, and a new chair was founded at Liverpool. Subsequently, two personal chairs were conferred, at Birmingham and Newcastle, and more lecturers appointed.[13] At the end of the war, there were about 40 experienced forensic pathologists practising virtually full-time,[14] and British forensic medicine was represented by several men of international distinction, with Smith and Glaister in Scotland, Keith Simpson, Donald Teare and Francis Camps in London, all with an apparently firm base in medical schools.

The old world of the heroic medical detective was fast disappearing, as new techniques made it impossible for any one man to comprehend the whole range of forensic medicine and science. Glaister and Smith still enjoyed giving a dramatic performance in the courtroom, but they knew how much their discipline depended on the work of less visible scientists. Glaister himself apparently did not regret the passing of the hand-to-hand combats, as he wrote in 1952:

> For long enough a tendency to rivalry and competition within our ranks has exercised a rather disintegrating influence on proper co-ordination and unity, [leading to] tolerance of unsatisfactory working conditions, of inadequate

remuneration, and of other factors whch would not have been accepted for a moment by those practising other branches of medicine...[15]

One event in particular created a profound impression on all the medical experts, and confirmed the value of an institutional base rather than free-lance work. In December 1947, Sir Bernard Spilsbury committed suicide in his laboratory. He was in his seventy-first year. His health was failing after a stroke; but with only a nominal attachment to a medical school, and no pension, he could not afford to retire. He continued with his court work and the coroners' autopsies at two guineas a time until he knew that he could no longer cope. Spilsbury, a cold and solitary man, had inspired little affection amongst his colleagues in forensic medicine, but the manner of his death was a tragedy exposing all the deficiencies of the system in which he worked.[16] Furthermore, although he left a popular reputation bordering on myth, there was no legacy of scholarship. The long-promised text on forensic medicine remained unwritten, for he could not spare the time from his routine cases. A place in a hospital or university team clearly had its advantages.

Yet at the very time that demand was rising, other upheavals inadvertently threatened the university base of forensic medicine. Both political parties made wartime promises to reform the health service after the war, and the Ministry of Health began a massive survey of the nation's hospitals and medical education. In 1944 a committee chaired by Sir William Goodenough reported on the medical schools, recommending that medical education be confined to the universities, and suggesting a national curriculum to take account of modern needs. The Committee intended to remedy many long-standing defects of medical education, but its view of forensic medicine was curt. Although Bernard Spilsbury, Sydney Smith and Andrew Allison gave evidence in various capacities, the report merely commented:

> In some medical schools the amount of instruction given to medical students on forensic medicine seems excessive having regard to the needs of general practice.[17]

At the time, the threat to the position of forensic medicine seemed vague, and in 1947 the General Medical Council reaffirmed the importance of forensic medicine in medical education.[18] The new National Health Service, however, offered no secure home for forensic medicine. Bevan's compromise with the medical profession was particularly favourable for hospital consultants, and the clinical staff of university medical schools had their salaries jointly funded by the universities and the NHS. Forensic medicine did not receive these benefits since its teachers did not have clinical posts: medico-legal experts in the universities were in a less secure position than the hospital pathologists, and still depended on fees from outside work.

Glaister resented the government's apparent willingness to leave forensic pathology to the voluntary efforts of hospital pathologists. NHS pathologists had a secure, pensionable, salary which they could supplement with Crown work: the forensic pathologists, by contrast, relied on fees which were not pensionable to make up their incomes.[19] Unlike other branches of medicine, forensic medicine remained particularly dependent on the goodwill and financial support of the universities. Glaister was anxious about this neglect of his subject, particularly the lack of a career structure, and accurately predicted that suitable recruits would be hard to find.[20] In 1947 he tried to set up his postgraduate course, with co-operation from the City Analyst and the police laboratory. The Corporation and the procurator fiscal approved, as they felt 'it would make available to both the Crown and the Defence,... a larger number of doctors with the necessary experience to apply medical knowledge in the forensic sphere.'[21] Glaister donated his collection of hairs to the police museum, partly as a friendly gesture, and partly, perhaps, to indicate that this type of work would no longer be the task of doctors. But no funds were available in Britain for postgraduate training in forensic medicine, and the scheme did not develop. Most of Glaister's postgraduate students came from overseas and were financed by governments wishing to improve their own forensic services.

Nevertheless, Glaister's empire expanded a little. In 1947, St Mungo's medical school was absorbed into the University of Glasgow, and Andrew Allison came back to the forensic medicine department as emeritus professor: he lectured to the department's class at the Royal Infirmary until he retired in 1953.[22] Also in 1947 came a new recruit, Edgar Rentoul, recently demobbed after outstanding medical service in Burma. Before the war, Rentoul's family came to think of him as a perpetual student, because he graduated first in law and then, in 1939, in medicine. In 1947, so the story goes, he was wandering rather hopefully around the university looking for some kind of employment, and, on passing the door of the forensic medicine department, decided to look in on his old teacher. Glaister took him on as an assistant at £400 a year, and he proved a popular choice. Handsome and affable, Rentoul was an amiable foil to the rather prickly Glaister. He became Glaister's 'second doctor', and they worked together on murder cases and other serious crimes throughout Scotland. After a while, Rentoul began to carry the heavier load of work for the fiscal, as Glaister tended to withdraw himself unless his services were specially required.

Although Glaister was not able to realise his dream of heading a medico-legal institute, he took a decision which led to his department becoming a joint enterprise between doctors and scientists. Wartime research opened up many new areas of science: nuclear physics was one of the most exciting, and scientists in many countries began to investigate its peaceful applications. Glaister saw the steady movement of forensic science away from medical experts into the hands of other specialists, but this did not prevent him from encouraging research into new techniques which he could no longer carry out himself.

In 1954, Glaister was approached by Dr John Lenihan, then working in the Regional Physics Department of the Western Regional Hospital Board, who suggested that the new techniques in activation analysis might also be applied to forensic medicine. Activation analysis, which uses nuclear methods to identify the component parts of any substance, depends on the fact that many elements become radioactive when bombarded with neutrons inside a

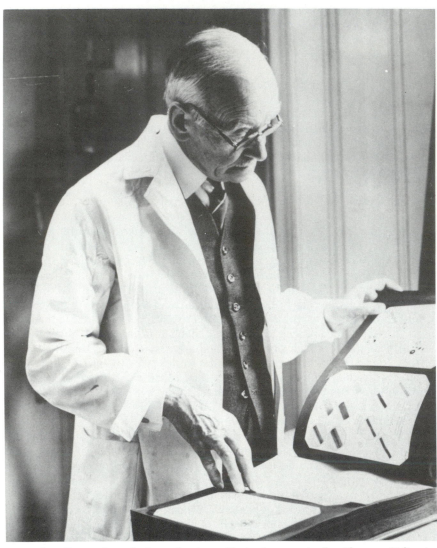

18   John Glaister Jr with the collection of hairs he gave to the Glasgow Police in
1947 (GP)

nuclear reactor. Each radioactive isotope produced in this way emits its own distinctive radiation, capable of identification and measurement—originally with Geiger counters, but now with more sophisticated electronic devices. Activation analysis is, for many elements, remarkably sensitive and has the added advantage (important when minute amounts of an element are sought) of freedom from contamination by laboratory reagents, which is always a danger in traditional methods of chemical analysis. Lenihan hoped to improve the new techniques and to put them to biological uses: activation analysis, he said later, was 'a solution in search of problems.'[23]

The irradiation of biological material in a living person was dangerous, and Lenihan considered identifying toxins which penetrated into detachable parts of the body, such as the hair. Arsenic and other mineral poisons, which were known to enter the hair rapidly, were obvious examples, and Glaister, with a family interest in arsenic and a personal interest in hair, was immediately attracted to the project. The Medical Research Council supplied finance, Glaister provided space in his laboratory, and a young graduate chemist, Hamilton Smith, was employed to work on activation analysis, with special reference to arsenic. (Glaister was pleased to have Smith's services, and used him as a general problem solver in other matters as well.)

Lenihan and Smith had first to estimate the normal occurrence of arsenic in human hair: this was difficult to achieve by chemical means because large quantities of hair were required. Activation analysis could be performed on small amounts of hair, pulled out by the roots, and, by measuring the concentration of arsenic along the length of the hair, the regularity of its ingestion could be measured. A large group of volunteers donated hair, and the experimenters were surprised to find that one group of female volunteers from a local hospital had alarmingly high levels of arsenic in their hair: the reason for this was traced to the women's frugal habit of using hospital detergent to wash their hair. The sulphuric acid used in the manufacture of this detergent had been made by the lead chamber process, in which contamination by arsenic (present as an impurity in one of the raw materials) has long been known. The manufacturers of the detergent immediately changed their suppliers of sulphuric acid.[24]

Although it was known that arsenic passes fairly rapidly into the hair, it was difficult to measure the time of absorption precisely. Lenihan and Smith proved, with the aid of intrepid volunteers, that arsenic would appear in hair very rapidly. Smith refined the technique to achieve a thousandfold improvement in sensitivity over previously available techniques and could analyse 50 samples a day; by these means he was able to use the hair as a 'calendar,' to chart the daily ingestion of arsenic, and later, of other dangerous substances.[25] A useful case history was presented to Lenihan for analysis: a patient with the classical signs of chronic arsenical poisoning had insisted on taking for 12 years an old-fashioned medicine containing heroic quantities of arsenic. His regular doses were mapped out in his hair.[26]

Lenihan and Smith originally thought that research on arsenic in the hair might reveal a link between cigarette smoking and cancer, since some of the cigarettes of the time contained relatively high levels of arsenic. Experiments on the hair of smokers and non-smokers, however, produced no appreciable difference in arsenic content. Although industrial and environmental poisonings were uppermost in the researchers' minds, their work suddenly became famous for unexpected reasons.

In 1961, Hamilton Smith was sent a small sample of hair from an unknown subject, and, on analysing it, detected arsenic at well above the concentration normally found. The subject was revealed to be the Emperor Napoleon, and the hair had probably been cut from his head immmediately after his death in exile on St Helena. Locks from the deceased emperor had been despatched to a number of his admirers, who preserved them reverently, and this particular relic was sent to Smith by a Swedish dentist, Dr Sten Forshufvud. Forshufvud and Smith published their findings in *Nature*, linking the suggestion of arsenical poisoning to the well-charted symptoms of Napoleon's last illness.[27] The article caused a sensation, and Hamilton Smith was amused at the passion it aroused amongst Napoleon scholars, both amateur and professional, who sent him many intemperate letters. The first article led to the acquisition of some longer strands of Napoleon's hair, from a well-attested source, confirming that Napoleon had received regular doses of arsenic for some time. Several more samples of Napoleon's hair arrived, all indicating arsenic, and including one sample dating from before his exile.[28] The authors, of course, could give no conclusive explanation for Napoleon's consumption of arsenic, and speculations included accidental poisoning from medicines, arsenical wallpaper, and (inevitably) homicide by his British captors.

The articles on Napoleon received such wide publicity that Smith became an involuntary historical analyst, and was sent hair from long-dead persons known and unknown. A Romano-British pigtail from near Dorchester revealed no disturbing elements; a medieval head from Sweetheart Abbey had substantial amounts of mercury in the hair only; King Charles II appeared to have been exposed to dangerous levels of mercury—a result of reckless scientific experiments?—and Robert Burns also revealed a high, though not dangerous, level of mercury absorption, possibly from over-prescription for liver disease.[29] As Lenihan said, these findings did not establish new historical theories, but demonstrated that 'scientific methods can be used to help the pathologist, even when the subject has been dead for more than a century.'[30]

Smith and Lenihan worked with the department of forensic medicine on a number of cases, and Smith joined the department, first as a research fellow and then, in 1964, as a lecturer. He was the first member of the department to be qualified in science rather than medicine. Toxicology was now a scientific, not a medical discipline, but Glaister had provided the foundation for the modern department, a partnership between doctors and scientists. Lenihan and Smith, with colleagues from clinical departments, continued their collaboration, and Smith worked on the detection of other dangerous substances in the body, including mercury and antimony. Many industrial poisons could be traced by their presence in hair, skin and nails. In particular, Smith and a colleague from the dental school challenged the received wisdom that dentists and their assistants were in no danger from their constant work with mercury in the preparation of fillings. On the contrary, dental workers had abnormal amounts of mercury in both hair and nails, warning of the danger of chronic poisoning.[31]

Like the health service, the universities also grew in the 1950s. Having given up territory to Public Health, the forensic medicine department was now threatened by the expansion of biochemistry. Glaister failed to retrieve the accommodation lost by the department when his father retired; instead the department moved into 8 University Gardens in 1955. The Coats family house, owned by an unbroken line of professors since 1918, was bought by the university for £3,250.[32] It was hardly purpose-built accommodation, but very grand. Structural alterations were made for the laboratory, and an animal house constructed at the back for the bad-tempered rabbits who provided blood for serological tests.

The university also provided the new department with more modern equipment, for much of its apparatus dated from 1932 when the younger Glaister took the chair. Old-fashioned equipment made heavy demands on both doctors and technicians, especially in intensive cases like Betty Alexander's. In the processing of human tissue for forensic examination under the microscope, the fluids bathing the tissue had to be changed regularly. At that time, preparation took up to ten days, and the fluids were changed every four hours. This was difficult for the technical staff, who faced coming into the department out of office hours, or making alternative arrangements. It was not unknown for histological processes of this kind to be carried out in temporary forensic laboratories at home, or even at social gatherings. In the freshly equipped department, a new automatic carousel, programmed by punch cards, took over this work. When Glaister first began to split hairs, he used razors which had to be sharpened laboriously on stones: the new microtomes needed no such care. Technicians in those days were trained in glassblowing, and most scientific departments could still make their own pipettes and test tubes as required.

Glaister occupied a majestic room with an imposing marble fireplace, and, always careful of his health, kept a thermometer to monitor the temperature. He also liked the staff to be lined up for their orders when he arrived in the morning. On cold Monday mornings, there was a problem if the cleaners had just lit the fire and the room had not reached the required warmth. When Glaister was seen getting out of his car, a resourceful technician would breathe heavily on the thermometer to bring it up to scratch, so that when the great man entered and checked it, he would nod approvingly.

As far as the medical members of the department were concerned, if guns had been a problem in the 1940s, then vehicles were the problem for the 1950s. Glaister was used to being called to examine vehicles for bloodstains, and occasionally for hair. In 1950, injuries from a car were the main point of the medico-legal evidence when James Robertson, a Glasgow police constable, was arrested for the murder of Catherine McCluskey.

Catherine McCluskey was 40 years of age, and the unmarried mother of two children. She was found dead near the junction of Prospecthill Road and Aikenhead Road, apparently the victim of a hit-and-run driver. The policeman first on the scene, however, was experienced in road traffic accidents, and became suspicious, firstly because he saw no sign of broken glass or any other debris from a car; and secondly, because there were *two* sets of wheel marks under the body, apparently going in opposite directions.[33] An indeterminate mark between the wheel marks might have been caused by a body being dragged along beneath a car. James Robertson, a 33-year old policeman, was supposedly on duty at the time of the death, but had left his beat, telling his colleague that he was 'off to see a blonde.' Shortly afterwards, he was seen driving a car with Catherine McCluskey as passenger.

Robertson was arrested, and admitted to causing the woman's death accidentally. This was his account of events. He knew Catherine McCluskey slightly, and gave her a lift when he saw her in the street: she was being turned out of her flat, and quarrelled with Robertson because he refused to take her to a friend's house in Neilston. He put her out of the car, but then changed his mind, and reversed back to where he left her. He felt no bump, but the noise from the exhaust sounded odd, so he stopped and got out, and found her body trapped under the car. In a panic, he tried unsuccessfully to pull her out, then drove backwards and forwards for a few yards until the body was free.

Other circumstances did not help Robertson. The car was a stolen one (which he said he had found abandoned), and he had changed its number plate. He also had a radio and a number of car license books, also stolen, and a heavy rubber truncheon, not of regulation issue.

Andrew Allison and James Imrie performed the post-mortem, but when the fiscal realised that forensic evidence would be vital, he also called Glaister and Walter Weir, pathologist at the Royal Alexandra Hospital in Paisley. Even with a medical team of this size, the evidence took many days to sift. Glaister mulled over the post-mortem report and the detailed police reports on the state of the car. He made numerous tests, matching Catherine McCluskey's dyed blonde hair to the hair found under the car, and examining the pattern of bloodstains on the wheels and under the car. He typed the bloodstains on the woman's clothes, and tested Robertson's clothes, and the truncheon, for blood. The benzidene test gave a positive result on the truncheon, but there was not enough staining for a more conclusive test; Robertson's clothes had no bloodstains, which rather contradicted his story of how he tried to free the body from the car. Glaister had long conferences with Allison and Imrie, and he also crawled around under the car, and got a policewoman to simulate the body, in order to work out how the injuries were sustained.[34] The case kept Glaister occupied almost full-time from 7 August until 8 September, and the fiscal also requested him to stay in court throughout the trial.

The prosecution's case relied heavily on the medical evidence. Catherine McCluskey had no injuries to the front of her legs, as would be expected after impact with the bumper of a car; but the inner parts of the knees had been badly gouged. The car wheels had passed over her neck, chest and pelvis, causing gross injuries. The car itself showed no signs of damage, except for a slight dent on the back bumper. Walter Weir prepared slides of cells from the scalp wounds and the knees: the pathologists agreed that the scalp wounds were caused before death, the leg wounds after death. Glaister argued in court that Catherine McCluskey must have been lying in a relaxed position in the road when the car hit her: she had been hit while the car was driving at considerable speed, and it then turned around and ran over her again. Why was she lying in the road? It was possible that she had been knocked unconscious (possibly with the truncheon), before the car was driven over her.

Although John Cameron, for the defence, argued manfully that Catherine McCluskey could have been lying in the road for a variety of reasons, the jury found Robertson guilty and he was hung. He would not admit that he had any connection with Catherine McCluskey, although her friends said they had seen him with her, and the prosecution tried to establish that he was in fact the father of her younger child, and paying her maintenance for it. This would have given her the power to threaten both his marriage and his career. Glaister spent 149 hours on the case, and was paid a fee of £187 19s. 0d. He must have relied on fees from big cases like this and Betty Alexander's (£126 for 110 hours), to supplement his not over-generous university salary.[35]

The department also worked on more common problems of road traffic, such as testing urine samples of drivers arrested for being unfit to drive. Rentoul became interested in the whole question of drunken drivers. Although drunken driving was an offence, there was, as all the forensic medicine textbooks admitted, no legal definition of 'drunk'. Medico-legal thinking on drunkenness was effectively summed up in the memorable verses Frank Martin used to recite to his students:

> He is not drunk, who, on the floor,
> Can still sit up and ask for more;
> But drunk is he who passive lies,
> And from the floor he cannot rise.[36]

Although alcohol in the blood and urine could be detected, there was no legal definition of an upper limit, nor could drivers be required to take a blood test. A driver could be charged only if he were proved to be incapable of handling the vehicle; hence the BMA's criteria for drunkenness, laid down in 1927 and revised from time to time, consisted of such matters as the driver's general manner, the state of his clothes, the appearance of his conjunctiva and of his tongue, pupil reaction, smell of alcohol on the breath, slurred speech, general co-ordination (as in picking up coins from the floor), memory, and hiccoughs.[37] None of this provided very solid evidence.

Edgar Rentoul and Hamilton Smith, together with Richard Beavers, the senior technician in the department, conducted further experiments on consumption of alcohol and its implications for road traffic offences. They noted the well-known deficiencies of the several Road Traffic Acts. An Act of 1960 allowed a conviction for drunken driving only if the driver had no 'proper control' over the vehicle. Since 'proper control' was impossible to define, the police normally arrested only those whose behaviour was severely impaired by drink—yet many drivers who showed less obvious signs of drunkenness had taken enough alcohol to be a danger to the public. The Road Traffic Act of 1962 set no limit to the amount of alcohol permissable in blood, but required that courts take account of the amount of alcohol in blood and urine. Drivers could refuse to give blood or urine samples, but this would tell against them in court.

The experiments were conducted with twenty volunteers; each drank 10 oz. of whisky in times varying from five to fifteen minutes. (The authors noted that 'the number of people who are prepared to drink ten ounces of whisky in a short time is surprisingly limited...no one showed any sign of exhilaration or ebullience.'[38]) Each volunteer was observed for four hours or more, and subjected to the standard police tests at regular intervals, as well as a test of their reaction time. Urine samples were also taken every hour. The results confirmed the unreliability of the usual police tests, such as walking a line or picking up coins. The authors measured reaction times, first by using an electronic counter in which the subject pressed a button as soon as he saw a light come on: then they invented a much cheaper version, in which the subject had to catch a broom handle as soon as it began to fall vertically through two holes. Reaction time was measured from a scale on the broom handle, according to the formula for estimating distance travelled by a falling body. As expected, the physical tests showed enormous individual variations; some could walk the line without difficulty, others were unable to walk at all. Nor was there any relationship between alcohol concentration in the urine and ability to perform physical tests. The authors recommended an absolute, if arbitrary, definition of being unfit to drive a vehicle: and suggested 100 milligrammes of alcohol to 100 millilitres of urine. It took some time, however, for the law to catch up with the recommendations of the experts. It was not until Barbara Castle's introduction of a compulsory breathalyser test in 1967, that the law established that 80 mg per 100 ml of alcohol in blood was as much as any driver should be allowed.

Rentoul provided a service to defence lawyers in analysing blood and urine for alcohol, but his work in serology also involved him in paternity cases. After Karl Landsteiner first reported on the existence of the blood groups in 1900, intensive research elaborated his findings. It was soon suggested that blood groups were subject to Mendelian laws of inheritance, and by 1924, the method of transmission was known.[39] The first groups to be discovered were A,B,AB and O, and in 1928, Landsteiner and Levine added two independent blood types, M and N. Tests for the MN system were more difficult to perform, and required much skill, as well as completely reliable sera. Rentoul carried out many such tests with Dr John Wallace, an expert in serology, and they gave evidence in civil cases, police work, and paternity suits. Most of their cases concerned fathers reluctant to pay maintenance, but they were also drawn into a case unique in Scottish legal history, when they gave evidence supporting a mother who tried to bastardise her child in order to gain custody. The woman married three weeks after the birth of her

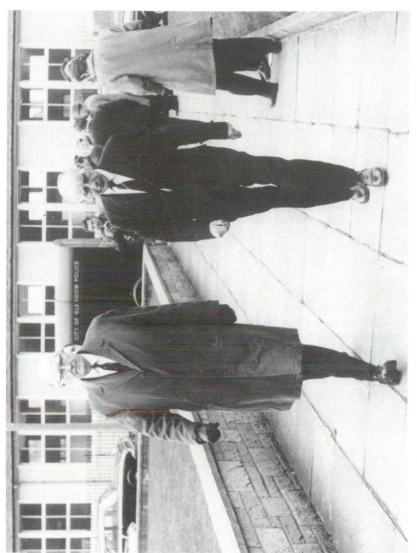

19   Edgar Rentoul (left) and James Imrie arriving at a murder scene in 1968 (Courtesy *Glasgow Herald* and *Evening Times*)

child; her husband believed himself to the the father, and under Scots law the marriage made the baby legitimate. The couple divorced before long on the grounds of the wife's adultery, and both remarried, though the husband kept custody of the child. His sister brought it up and became very attached to it. After her remarriage, the mother tried to get custody of the child by the novel claim that her former husband was not its father: she named instead a Polish serviceman who could not be traced. Rentoul and Wallace carried out the blood tests, and found that the ABO and rhesus tests offered no conclusive evidence. On the basis of the MN test, however, they argued that the chances of the former husband being the child's father were 100,000 against. The defence contended that the MN test was not reliable because of the possibility of a genetical mutation between generations, (such mutations do occur regularly but infrequently) and the difficulty of detecting a factor in blood known as N_2. It was accepted that the experts knew of these problems, and had carried out the tests with extreme care. Lord Wheatley's judgment was in favour of the mother, though he did not base it entirely on the medical evidence:

> Where...such evidence is based on scientific medical research which is always on the move in one direction or another, and the possibility of further development or discovery cannot be ignored...the Court should have regard to the non-medical evidence in the case to see to what extent the scientific evidence is confirmed or confuted by such other evidence.[40]

The dispossessed father appealed against this decision, and, to the great surprise of the expert witnesses, the court reversed the original decision and accepted that the child was his. The appeal court, having rejected evidence about the mysterious Polish serviceman, refused to accept that the relatively complicated blood testing technique was adequate evidence on its own. In addition, the father argued that he had voluntarily submitted to a blood test without realising that it could not prove his paternity, but only disprove it.[41] As in Glaister's early work with precipitin tests, the courts were always cautious in accepting new techniques. For some time, experts regarded the judgment as quite unreasonable, but more recent work, which has identified a rare Mg factor in the blood, increases the possibility that the putatitive father's claim was just.[42]

The department of forensic medicine also kept students abreast of new methods by regularly producing new editions of Glaister's *Medical Jurisprudence*. Rentoul gave Glaister legal advice for the 9th edition in 1950, and became co-author of subsequent editions, first with Glaister and then with Hamilton Smith after Glaister retired. The luxuriant anecdotes of Glaister senior were pruned away, the photographs in colour were an even harder test for weak stomachs, and the text became more functional, no doubt to the students' relief.

In his prime, the younger Glaister was also a dynamic lecturer, and the lecture-room was crammed in spite of the early hour. No paper aeroplanes swirled around his head—the traditional fate of Glasgow professors who failed to command the students' attention. The Bedellus locked the door of the lecture theatre promptly at 9 a.m., and no latecomer was admitted. Glaister, like his father, believed in visual aids, and was one of the first lecturers in medicine to use coloured slides. He used the Ruxton case and several of his wartime investigations to illustrate techniques in forensic medicine, and employed the dramatic device (frowned on by safety experts, but a favourite at that time of lecturers in forensic medicine), of pulling out a gun from his briefcase and pointing it at the audience. In Glaister's classes, the long-suffering Bedellus was the target, but the tactic never failed to keep the students awake during a discussion of entrance and exit wounds. Glaister continued his father's practice of taking small groups of students to hear him give evidence in court. His courtroom technique became as highly polished as an actor's performance, and he forced the lawyers to take the evidence at his pace, slowing them down, if necessary, by much cleaning of his glasses and very deliberate consultation of his notes. For most of the students, his teaching was a guide to their legal responsibilities in general practice: there was no obvious career path into forensic medicine. Yet one of the graduates of the 1950s briefly became a lecturer in pathology and worked with Rentoul: the path then led to Francis Camps' department at the London Hospital, and to a distinguished career in forensic medicine. This was Professor J.M. ('Taffy') Cameron, now professor of Forensic Medicine in the University of London.

Inevitably, 'Young John' became 'Old John' in his turn, a small but formidable figure in dignified pin-stripes, alarming to students and junior colleagues, but an entertaining companion in his own circles. It is pleasing to record that he finally achieved some of his early ambition of reaching a wider audience. He was always interested in popularising forensic medicine, and in 1949 he met Erle Stanley Gardner, the famous creator of Perry Mason. They became friends and corresponded regularly: Gardner admired Glaister's *Medical Jurisprudence* and his work on the Ruxton case; while Glaister himself decided to try his hand at detective fiction. In co-operation with the Scottish novelist Maurice Lindsay, he wrote a novel entitled *Broke the Fair Music,* which seems, from the fragments which survive in his papers, to have been a rather indigestible mixture of fey rural romanticism and grimly realistic medical detection. In spite of Gardner's assistance, Glaister was not able to find a publisher for his novel, but their friendship survived the setback, and in 1964 Gardner dedicated to Glaister his latest murder mystery, *The Case of the Horrified Heirs*, and sent him the certificated first copy off the press.

Glaister had less difficulty with non-fiction, and in 1954 published a book on famous poisoning cases, entitled *The Power of Poison*, though this too was not a commercial success. He retired in 1962, and set to work on his memoirs: this time he took the wise precaution of enlisting the help of a young journalist, William Knox, to prepare them for publication as *Final Diagnosis* (1964). Glaister's life was much more interesting than his fiction, and is still very readable. In return, Bill Knox found that his discussions with Glaister gave him an introductory course on forensic medicine, useful for his own successful career as a crime novelist.

Glaister also achieved success in a new medium which gave him enormous

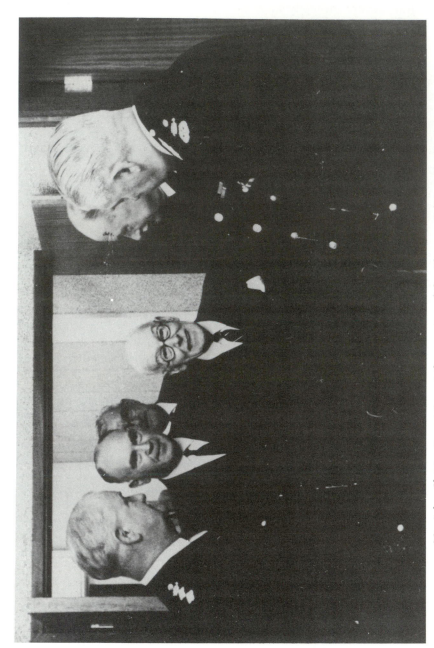

20   John Glaister Jr arriving at the opening of the Glasgow Police Scientific Laboratories in 1968 (GP)

pleasure. The first attempt failed: in 1965, STV screened four episodes of a series called *Glaister*, which took up his familiar cases but was rather uneasily pitched between drama and documentary; also, as the cases were well known, they lacked suspense. Glaister's nephew, Gerard Glaister, then produced a BBC series entitled *The Expert*, loosely based on Glaister's character and cases, but with a fictional approach. With a fine actor, Marius Goring, in the leading role, it was very popular, and further series were made. Goring stayed with the Glaisters to watch the professor's mannerisms and gain a closer insight into the way he worked. Glaister gave the series technical advice and extra material; he also enjoyed the opportunity to return to the theatrical atmosphere he had loved as a young man. Had he been born at a later date, he would doubtless have become a television personality in his own right: as it was, he made only one appearance, with great poise.

The press followed his movements with relish, as they had his father's, and when he retired the *Daily Herald* conferred on him the title he would have least appreciated, 'The Sir Bernard Spilsbury of Scotland'.[43] In 1968 he was an honoured guest at the opening of the new forensic laboratory of the City of Glasgow police, and under the headline THE CRIME BUSTERS, the *Scottish Daily Express* reported GLAISTER IS THERE; GLAISTER LOOKS IN ON SCIENCE 'TECS.[44]

Glaister died in October 1971, aged 79. When his career began, the courts would barely accept that he could distinguish human from animal blood: when it ended, forensic techniques were changing so rapidly that the courts rarely challenged expert opinion, except on the interpretation of evidence. In the process, however, the medical expert could no longer claim authority over the province of the chemist, the biologist, or the psychiatrist; his boundaries had constantly to be redrawn. The growing danger was that the separate services would lack cohesion, as Sydney Smith had said in 1951:

> The present-day problem is largely one of providing establishments or institutes where a combination of these specialists can suitably operate as a team when necessary. Different countries have tackled the problem in different ways, and... it might be remarked that the arrangements in Britain are not yet ideal.[45]

Smith, Spilsbury and the Glaisters hoped in vain for medico-legal institutes with all the forensic services under one roof: instead, the system was fragmented between the universities, the hospitals, and the police laboratories. Glaister was one of the last of the versatile medical detectives. In his later years he accepted benignly the arrival of the new forensic scientists with degrees in chemistry or biology, for he was secure in the knowledge that courts still gave the greater respect to the confident medical expert with so many famous cases behind him. The name of Glaister had been in the forefront of Scottish forensic medicine for 64 years: their successors would have to work within a different order.

CHAPTER SEVEN

A Modern Department

Glaister's retirement from the regius chair in 1962 immediately exposed some of the difficulties confronting forensic medicine in Scotland. The regius chair in Edinburgh also stood empty. Douglas Kerr, Sydney Smith's successor, died in 1960, and there was no regius professor until 1973, when John Kenyon Mason was appointed. Both universities confronted the same questions: how to define the professor's role in an age of specialisation, and whether other branches of medical education had a stronger claim to finance.

Glaister's gloomy predictions on the future of forensic medicine appeared entirely justified. The prosperity of the British economy encouraged a great expansion of the NHS, particularly the hospital services. Pathology itself was expanding and becoming more specialised in the large hospital laboratories: it offered a secure career and the opportunity for research into many interesting problems. The Glaisters termed themselves 'medico-legists', not 'forensic pathologists'. The old title reflected their wide interests in law and medicine, but by the time the younger Glaister retired, it was becoming more accurate to use the modern, and more specialised term. A young doctor interested in pathology now had a wide choice of careers, but forensic pathology offered few opportunities and little security.

In addition, some members of the Glasgow medical faculty thought that forensic medicine took up too much time in an increasingly crowded curriculum. It was argued that the numbers of lectures in forensic medicine should be much reduced, 'to avoid students being burdened with knowledge that is today the province of specialists', and that much of it should be confined to postgraduates.[1] The Law faculty considered whether studies in criminology might be of more use to their own students:[2] forensic medicine had not been compulsory for the Bachelor of Law degree since 1954, and was now one of a range of options.

Representatives from Edinburgh and Glasgow universities discussed the future of forensic medicine, and the Crown Office took much interest in the negotiations. Glasgow decided to advertise for a professor who would continue the tradition of serving the needs of the city. But the advertised salary of £2,900 was considerably below the expectations of senior pathologists with both university and clinical posts. James Imrie was interested in the chair, but was only eight years from retirement, and the police made it clear that they did not wish to lose him.

Few candidates appeared, and the university tried head-hunting. But some of the most suitable candidates indicated that the salary was lower than they would accept; the university had to think again; and the regius chair was then offered with a salary at clinical level, and an honorary consultancy in the Western Infirmary.[3] In return for this higher, and pensionable, salary, the bulk of the fees from outside work would go to the university and not to the professor. The Crown Office had no power to offer any financial help, but was anxious, since both regius chairs were empty, to safeguard 'the high scientific medical opinion' which was 'most desirable in the more difficult cases with which the procurator fiscal had to deal.'[4] The chair was accepted by Gilbert Forbes, then Reader in charge of the department of forensic medicine at the University of Sheffield, Pathologist to the City of Sheffield Police, and Home Office pathologist for South Yorkshire. Apart from his long experience in the field, he had the additional advantages of being a Scotsman, and a graduate of the University of Glasgow.

Gilbert Forbes was in his fifties at the time of his appointment, and had been in Sheffield since 1937. He was a wide ranging medico-legist of the old school, and, having been a police surgeon, was active in clinical forensic medicine—that is, he examined the living as well as the dead. In Sheffield he saw many victims of sexual crimes, and gave evidence on hairs, fibres, stains and serology as well as performing autopsies. The new professor, serious and bowler-hatted, was addicted to his work, and was soon heavily engaged in investigations for the fiscal. He started a campaign to persuade local authorities to improve the mortuaries outside Glasgow, some of which were in a disgusting condition. In one mortuary, the professor conducted post-mortems while standing in a large puddle. As Forbes' contemporary, Donald Teare, remarked about this time: 'few votes are caught by a stainless steel mortuary in comparison with a chromium plated ante-natal clinic.'[5] Gradually, several of the worst mortuaries were closed, and bodies brought to the better-equipped centres.

Like Rentoul, he undertook clinical work, and the department still had a room where victims of sexual abuse could be examined. Like the Glaisters, Professor Forbes also had an interest in work for insurance companies. He rarely relaxed, even at weekends, and expected everyone in the department to keep up with him. The staff could not believe that he had time for any recreation apart from cleaning his car.

Although Forbes hoped the department would expand, the number of pathologists remained at two during his tenure: Edgar Rentoul died in 1970 and was replaced by the department's first senior lecturer, Alan Watson, who, after a varied career including a medical mission in Zaire, had settled down as a Fellow of Queens' College, Cambridge, and consultant pathologist in Addenbrooke's hospital. Watson had a diploma in forensic pathology, and experience of working for the Coroner; he knew Glasgow well from a five-year attachment to the Western Infirmary and lectureship at the University. Now he succumbed to Professor Forbes' blandishments and decided to devote himself to forensic medicine.

The forensic pathologists remained a rare species, but toxicology expanded.

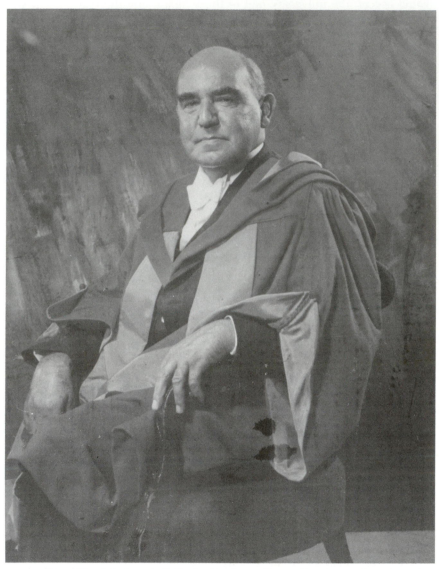

21   Gilbert Forbes, sixth Regius Professor (dept of forensic medicine)

Hamilton Smith set up a small analytical service, and by the late 1960s it was investigating about 500 cases a year. Among its first contracts was one from the the National Greyhound Racing Club for research into doping of racing greyhounds. It was not the department's first involvement with the dog track. The younger Glaister tested the hair of a champion racer, which, it was alleged, had been dyed and run under the false name of 'Black Aggie' in order to lengthen the odds. Armed with information from Regent's Park Zoo on the growth rate and moulting of dog hairs, Glaister found traces of the dye.[6]

Drugs are not metabolised in greyhounds in same way as in human beings, since greyhounds have virtually no fat. However, unlike athletes, greyhounds are rarely drugged to improve performance, since stimulants make their running erratic: but they may be doped—the canine equivalent of 'taking a dive'. The same effect can be achieved by giving them a meat pie or some milk, but this, unlike drugs, is easily seen by the veterinarians who examine them just before the race.

The National Greyhound Racing Club, responsible for the conduct of a leisure industry worth many millions, is a valuable though unusual supporter of academic research. Since the 1960s, the Club has regularly funded this research, which has implications also for drug detection in human subjects. Smith used the then new methods of thin-layer chromatography to test the greyhounds' urine: this had to be done very rapidly at the stadium in the hour before the race. The tests benefited the racing fraternity by effectively discouraging drug use. In return, Hamilton Smith had finance for better equipment and a regular supply of research students. Ultimately, as consultant toxicologist to the Club, Smith had an overview of some 50 analysts in 20 laboratories: where there is cause for suspicion, samples are still sent to the university laboratory.

The largest research project, however, was still in activation analysis, which aroused international interest. Once new techniques for biopsy were developed, activation analysis could identify trace elements in internal organs as well as hair and nails, and was particularly suitable for the tiny amounts of material produced in biopsy. Smith's work made it possible not only to detect abnormal quantities of certain elements in living tissue, but to determine the *normal* quantities more accurately.

Smith's laboratory complemented the work of the pathologists by testing for drugs and alcohol in dead bodies. The fiscals in the West of Scotland used this service increasingly: the beginnings were small, but the social problem of drugs rapidly increased the demand. The police laboratories had plenty of work in analysing suspicious substances, and so the complementary task of the university forensic scientists was to look for drugs and poisons in body tissue and body fluids. The laboratory served not only the fiscals, but hospitals, industry, and private individuals.

The toxicology work clearly required manpower, and Professor Forbes was able to appoint two more scientists, Dr John Oliver and Dr James Thorpe. Thorpe had a special interest in serology. The department also had the services of five technicians. Another sign of the break with the past was that the old medico-legal museum disappeared, and the elder Glaister's lovingly collected specimens were thrown out or banished to attics and cupboards under the stairs. Forbes was anxious to broaden the experience of his staff by sending them to busy departments elsewhere, and so Watson and Oliver spent some time in the office of the Chief Medical Examiner for New York, and Thorpe went to the 'Met' laboratories at Hendon.

Forbes, like his predecessors, seems to have yearned for an 'Institute of Forensic Medicine', to include not only pathology, but a wide range of services in toxicology, serology, clinical forensic medicine and even ballistics; and he argued that the university was its proper home:

> It is important that an institute should have the confidence of the public, and therefore it is better that it should be in a university and independent of the police. The public should know that the staff of the institute are impartial and that they can have access to them at any time when they desire help in criminal or civil matters.[7]

Forbes was not successful, however, in achieving further expansion, and in 1966, an entrepreneurial venture by Dr Francis Fish resulted in the establishment of a Forensic Science Unit at the University of Strathclyde, with particular strength in analytical chemistry, separation techniques and serology, as well as toxicology. Strathclyde concentrated on its postgraduate course in forensic science, and is one of the two universities in Britain offering this training.

Forensic science was burgeoning in Glasgow, though divided between the police and the two universities. As Forbes drew near his retirement, and with the Edinburgh chair still vacant, the problem of providing an adequate service in forensic pathology arose once again. The problem was not confined to Scotland, and finally aroused the attention of government. In 1960, Dr J D J Havard, with the encouragement of Sir Leon Radzinowicz, published a provocative book entitled *The Detection of Secret Homicide*. Havard traced the history of the coroner's inquest in England, and argued that it was in many respects unfitted for the detection of murder. He indicted the English medical schools for failing to teach forensic medicine adequately, for this led to ignorance among general practitioners, and lax practices in making out death certificates.[8] Since cremation was now a common practice, many more murders might remain undetected, with the forensic evidence destroyed, and Havard produced many examples of murders which had come to light accidentally, after all the legal formalities were over. Other research suggested that if a hospital doctor or general practitioner certified the cause of death, a post-mortem would confirm their findings in only 45% of cases.[9] The BMA followed this line of argument in its own report *Deaths in the Community* (1964), and in 1965 the Conservative government appointed a committee under Norman Brodrick, QC to investigate the whole subject of death certification and coroners.

The committee's report in 1971 concluded that these criticisms were alarmist, but nevertheless recommended a tightening of procedures in issuing death certificates. It was also anxious to have more autopsies, less for the detection of homicide than for increasing medical knowledge and improving national statistics on causes of death. This suggestion, which was likely to require the services of many more pathologists, was not acted on. Not only did economies in the NHS work against it, but the public would hardly have favoured more post-mortems for the sake of medical statistics, especially as most of the dead were elderly hospital patients.

The Brodrick Report argued that the Scottish system was in some ways less satisfactory than the English, for the fiscals tended to see autopsies as useful only if the findings might be needed in court. Hence in 1969, 27.4% of deaths in England, but only 16.1% of deaths in Scotland, resulted in an autopsy.[10] The Scottish system, being more centralised, was more consistent in its aim than the English, and more respectful of the wishes of relatives, but still left loopholes for undetected crime.

Against this background, and concerned about the future of the Scottish services in forensic pathology, the Scottish Home and Health Department in 1972 set up a joint working party with the Crown Office to investigate the state of forensic pathology in Scotland. It was chaired by John McCluskey QC, and then, on McCluskey's appointment as Solicitor General for Scotland in 1974, by S Bowen.[11] Gilbert Forbes was a member of this working party, which included representatives from the law, medicine, and the police.

The McCluskey report confronted the central problem squarely: although the services of forensic pathologists were essential to the purposes of the law, no-one had a duty to provide them. The police surgeons, who had once undertaken a wide range of services, were now fully occupied in clinical work. The Crown needed the pathologists, but its financial support went no further than paying a fee for each case. This was not sufficient security to attract doctors into forensic pathology as a career unless they had another source of income. In the larger centres of population, the universities and hospitals offered these services; in remoter areas, the general practitioners. The whole system was informal, depending on the departments of forensic medicine in the universities, and voluntary labour from hospital pathologists and general practitioners.

The McCluskey report was adamant that, as far as possible, only doctors with special training in forensic pathology should undertake work for the fiscals. But the pressure of work was becoming very heavy. The Universities could not afford to employ more forensic pathologists than were needed in the teaching of medical students; nor could the NHS hospitals be expected to permit their pathologists to spend large, and unpredictable, amounts of time working for the fiscal. Although hospital pathologists were the fiscals' main support in many parts of Scotland, hospitals had no formal commitment, and could not guarantee that their staff would always include a pathologist with an interest in medico-legal work.

For these reasons, the McCluskey report wished to consolidate forensic medicine in the four universities of Edinburgh, Glasgow, Aberdeen and Dundee.

Taking into account the important part that university departments of forensic medicine play in the development and provision of forensic pathology services, their involvement in training of both doctors and lawyers and the close working relationship which they have with the criminal authorities and the defence we felt that it would be logical to seek ways in which the present informal arrangement could be formalised and become the basis of a 'regional' service. To this end we would recommend that universities be invited to consider the possibility of their departments of forensic medicine assuming responsibility for the co-ordination on a regional basis of the forensic pathology service and also in playing a greater part in its provision. In making this recommendation we recognise that suitable financial arrangements will require to be made.[12]

Hospital pathologists would still have a part to play, especially in remote areas, but would be able to call on specialised services from the regional centres when necessary.[13] It was recommended that the Crown Office set up a national co-ordinating committee for forensic medicine, and that the heads of the university departments organise local committees of 'providers and users of the service.' The problem of training in forensic medicine could be solved if graduates training in pathology spent some time in a forensic medicine department or pathological laboratory to gain some experience.

Finance was the central issue. The report urged that forensic pathologists in the universities be paid salaries equivalent to their clinical colleagues (this was already the case in Glasgow, but not in all the universities), and that the Crown make a block grant to the universities instead of paying individual fees to the experts. The grant would also allow more staff to be appointed. The McCluskey report made no suggestion as to the amount of Crown subsidy to the universities. It left this decision to the 'national committee', but in fact this was never established. These recommendations, in spite of the rather vague financial directives, were in line with the ideas of many leading forensic pathologists in both England and Scotland.

In 1979, the Government approved these proposals, subject to the agreement of the universities.[14] Negotiations were slow: the universities were already in the toils of severe government economies, and were unable to commit themselves to long-term plans requiring much expenditure. The Civil Service, not to mention the NHS, were also under financial constraints.

Meanwhile, in Glasgow there was a new regime. Gilbert Forbes retired in 1974 and it was his successor who began the complicated negotiations with the Crown Office. The seventh Regius Professor was Arthur Harland, an enormous Ulsterman with a genial manner and buccaneering spirit. The road from the University of Belfast had taken him to hospitals in the USA, Canada and Jamaica, but since 1964 he had been in Glasgow, as senior lecturer in Pathology and consultant at the Western Infirmary. He was particularly experienced in the heart condition known as atheroma, but what he lacked in wide experience of medico-legal work he made up for by his intense interest in the scientific basis of forensic medicine. He had a passion for the most up-to-date equipment, and shortly after his arrival the department received its first mass spectrometer—a complex, computer-linked piece of equipment for identifying substances by bombarding them with a stream of electrons, which

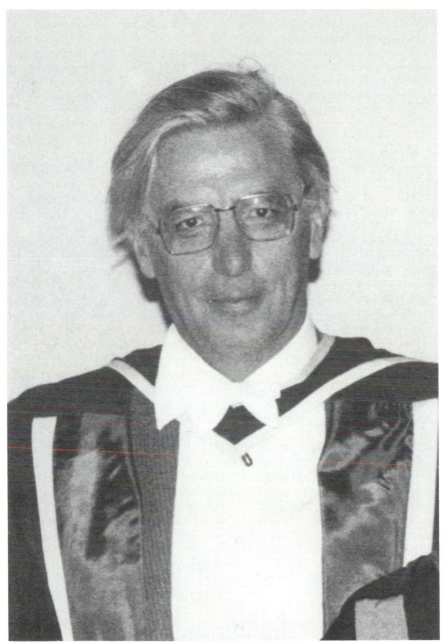

22   Arthur Harland, seventh Regius Professor (dept of forensic medicine)

break them down into charged fragments capable of separation and measurement.[15] The technical revolution permeated all aspects of the department's life, including an early replacement of typewriters by word-processors.

Harland was less interested in clinical work than in medical science, and the department undertook no more clinical examinations: the police surgeons, conversely, ceased to do autopsies. Nor did the department maintain its previous interests in hairs, fibres, or serology; James Thorpe took his serological expertise to the University of Strathclyde, and was replaced by Dr Robert Anderson, who was then a research fellow in the department. The new equipment was used in a project on fire deaths, begun by John Oliver and Alan Watson in the early 1970s, and in which most of the other members of the department subsequently became involved.

The fire deaths research showed the benefits of co-operation between pathologists and toxicologists.[16] Preliminary research by Oliver and Watson raised questions not only about the exact cause of death in fires, but why the victims had been unable to save themselves. Their joint investigation into the deaths of 36 adult victims of domestic fires revealed that alcohol and depressant drugs such as sleeping pills were present in 32 cases: they also argued that the chemical composition of fire smoke had not been adequately investigated.[17] There was need to compare laboratory research into the composition of smoke with samples taken from actual fires.

A large research project was funded by the Building Research Establishment Fire Research Station, to investigate the role of smoke and toxic gases in causing fire deaths. Between 1955 and 1978 fire deaths in the UK were rising, and the proportion of casualties due to smoke or fire gases was known to be an important factor. The Strathclyde region, unfortunately, was a good area for such studies, since the number of fire deaths—fifty or more a year—was 60% above the average rate for the UK. The Crown Office supported the research, directing the procurators fiscal to call the department's pathologists to perform all autopsies on victims of fire deaths. The toxicologists then carried out routine tests for drugs and alcohol, and special tests for other toxins which might have been inhaled.

Between 1976 and 1979, the department examined 199 victims of fire, but excluded from their statistics 17 deaths from suicide, traffic accident or homicide. Most fires broke out in the home; but there were also fatal accidents in furniture factories. Many bodies were so badly burned that it was not possible to tell whether the burns or some other factor had been the actual cause of death. However, 84% showed signs of respiratory injuries, indicating the possibility that they had died from inhaling toxic substances rather than from burns. The toxicologists then investigated further: they found signs of unusual cyanide levels in 12% of cases and carbon monoxide in 52%—both suggestive of inhalation of smoke.[18] Glasgow's notorious level of alcohol consumption (combined with heavy use of chip pans), led to more fires being started than in other parts of the country, but the team's findings gave empirical confirmation to the suspicion that smoke was the main reason for the growing numbers of fire deaths. This, and the work of other researchers, pointed towards the heavy smoke given off by the synthetics used in modern upholstery: it was not so much the toxicity of the smoke, but the fact that it soon rendered victims unconscious, which led to fatal results. This was a political problem, since economic interests were at stake, and the researchers at that time despaired of any action being taken to reduce fatalities: in 1987, however, after several incidents where whole families died as a result of smoke inhalation, the government finally decided to insist on the use of less dangerous material in upholstery.

Harland made changes in the department's teaching, accepting that forensic medicine as practised by the professionals was too specialised for the general education of undergraduates.[19] He noted with unease the steady decline of forensic medicine in British universities: the eight chairs of the immediate post-war period were reduced to three. In 1950 the General Medical Council dropped its requirement for a compulsory examination in medical jurisprudence for medical students, and in the 1970s only a few of the Scottish and Northern Irish universities insisted on it. By the 1980s, Glasgow and Belfast were the only universities to require it. Harland's predecessors used to teach their students how to conduct a post-mortem, and spent much time lecturing on violent death. The modern students, whether general practitioners or hospital doctors, would leave all this to the experts, and did not need detailed instruction.

Harland's response was to change the emphasis of the department's medical teaching 'to provide an understanding of doctors' legal obligations and of the legal hazards of medical practice.'[20] The department offered 44 lectures in forensic medicine to undergraduates in law, and 20 lectures in medical jurisprudence to the medical students.[21] Harland and Watson were also interested in keeping themselves, their students and colleagues up to date with legal changes as they affected the medical profession, and this led in 1975 to the appointment of a lawyer, Sheila McLean, to the department's staff. This broke with the previously masculine tradition of the academic staff. Sheila McLean was particularly interested in the impact of law and ethics on medicine, including such questions as medical negligence, patient consent and reproduction technology: she established a popular option within the honours school of the Law Faculty. The Ordinary Class for lawyers also increased in popularity, though it had less emphasis on forensic pathology and included short courses on forensic psychiatry and the uses of forensic science. Here the department was also able to draw on the expertise of other specialists from outside the university. The more specialised teaching was left for postgraduate students, and new degrees were offered, an M.Sc. in Medical Science (Forensic Medicine); an M.Sc. and diploma in Forensic Toxicology, and an LL.M.

Harland may have had cause to reflect, however, that the old justification for teaching forensic medicine to all medical students still had its points. General practitioners are often the first to examine a body, and must be alert to suspicious circumstances. A young Glasgow GP found this out to his embarrassment when he was called to issue a death certificate for an elderly member of the Pakistani community. The old gentleman, with a history of heart disease, was lying peacefully in bed in his pyjamas, though his head was covered. The young doctor, sensitive to what he presumed were the religious practices of the family, did not remove the head covering, but examined the body and issued a certificate of death from heart disease. Later, after members of the family became suspicious, it was revealed that the man had not died in bed, but in the street outside: he had been assaulted and robbed, and his head injuries were discovered only after the body had been flown to Pakistan for burial. Harland and Watson had to fly to Pakistan, arrange for an exhumation, and perform a post-mortem in somewhat unpleasant conditions.[22] A trial and conviction followed.

Meanwhile, the Crown Office continued negotiations with the four universities on the funding of forensic pathology. Aberdeen was the first to begin the new system, with Crown funds available to transfer two lecturers from the department of pathology into forensic medicine: the university then took responsibility for all fiscal autopsies in the Grampian region.[23] Negotiations with Glasgow University were largely complete by May 1983, and put the whole financial position of the department on a new footing. It was decided that the department should, in stages, take over the greater proportion of autopsies for the fiscal in the West of Scotland, and the staff be expanded to cope with this. The original aim was for the universities to undertake two-thirds of all autopsies for legal purposes, and for the hospital pathologists to undertake the rest. In practice, the fiscal also took advice from the forensic pathologists to summon hospital-based specialists such as neuro-pathologists or paediatric pathologists when necessary.

As a result of the negotiations, two pathologists were appointed with salaries supported by the Crown Office, which also made some contribution towards running costs. Dr John Clark came in 1984, and Dr Marie Cassidy in 1985: two further appointments are currently (1988) being arranged. At a time when the universities are painfully reducing their staff, the department of forensic medicine has been able to go against the current and expand its services to the city of Glasgow and the West of Scotland.

Arthur Harland died suddenly in 1985, before the new scheme came into full operation. He always took great interest in the history of his office, and it was he who first suggested that this book be written. His successor was Alan Watson, now the eighth Regius Professor of Forensic Medicine, and the first Englishman permitted to occupy the chair. In Harland's time, in recognition of the developing scientific service, the department's name changed to Forensic Medicine and Science.

The department presently consists of the eighth Regius Professor, the Professor of Toxicology (Hamilton Smith), two toxicologists, two forensic pathologists, with a further appointment in pathology already made and another to come, one lawyer and two part-time tutors in law. There are also five technicians, together with laboratory assistants, and the secretarial staff. There are also a number of research students—usually about five each year.

The authors had intended to end this history by describing the work of the present staff, and, with this in mind, asked each to provide an account of his, or her, research and other responsibilities. The response was such a daunting list of projects and learned publications, both in combination with one another

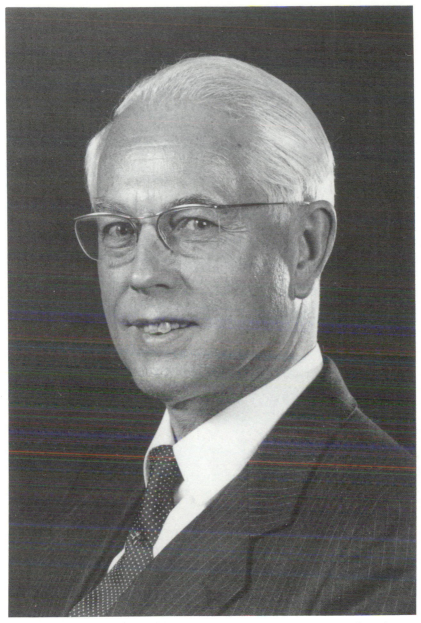

23   Alan Watson, eighth Regius Professor (dept of forensic medicine)

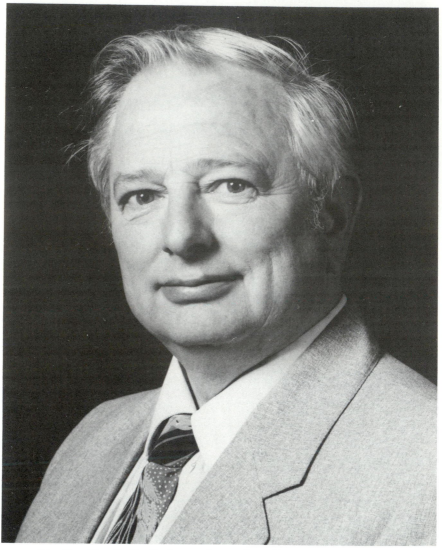

24 Hamilton Smith, Professor of Toxicology (dept of forensic medicine)

and with colleagues from outside the department, that it seemed impossible to list them all briefly, and invidious to select only a few. It is appropriate, therefore, to conclude this account of how a single, unwanted, professorship grew into such a considerable enterprise, by describing the daily routine of the modern department.

At the close of 1987 the department moved from 8 University Gardens and crossed back over University Avenue to a specially designed complex within the chemistry building, but separate from other departments for security reasons. The building bears an appropriate plaque to Joseph Black, the eighteenth-century polymath, who held sway in the university as chemist, anatomist, and professor of the Practice of Medicine. The move left many regrets for the 'old house' and some fears that its familial atmosphere might be lost. In the old building, information passed easily up and down the elegant mahogany staircase linking the department's four floors: in the more functional chemistry building, corridors link pathology and science on the ground floor. Communication is now horizontal rather than vertical. The department no longer handles bulky 'productions' like Dr Ruxton's bathtub, but police motorcyclists clad in brilliant fluorescent jackets are constantly arriving with samples for analysis.

The change in working conditions has been greatest for the scientists. Over the years the space available inside the old house was exploited to the full as the toxicology laboratories expanded. The battery of expensive equipment was lodged uneasily in rooms originally intended for domestic arrangements, from the maids' room to the laundry and the broom cupboards. This, one of the largest laboratories for forensic toxicology in Europe, with an international reputation, was cramped behind the facade of late Victorian splendour.

The laboratories in the new building are more suitable and spacious. The toxicological laboratories take fiscal, police and civil work. The volume of fiscal work has almost doubled in recent years. At the same time, the Strathclyde police, faced with ever-rising numbers of street drug offences, transferred their own post-mortem toxicology service to the department. For the same reasons, the police also discontinued drug identification in road traffic offences. This means that at present the department carries out all the forensic post-mortem toxicology analyses in this part of Scotland. Analysis under the Road Traffic Act of 1972 is divided between the police laboratory and the university, with the police conducting tests for alcohol in blood and urine, and the university toxicologists testing for drugs and, in defence cases, for alcohol. The toxicologists are all authorised analysts under the Road Traffic Acts.

Growing reliance on the breathalyser has reduced the number of defence cases which come to the department, since the police findings are less frequently challenged. In cases where the defence of post-accident consumption of alcohol is used (the so-called 'hip-flask' defence), the department receives

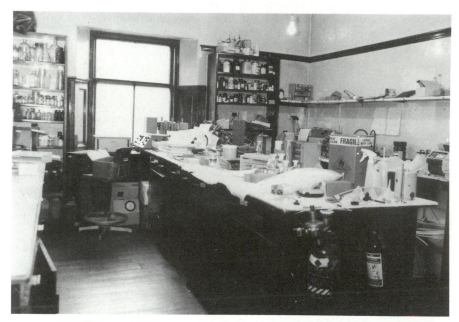

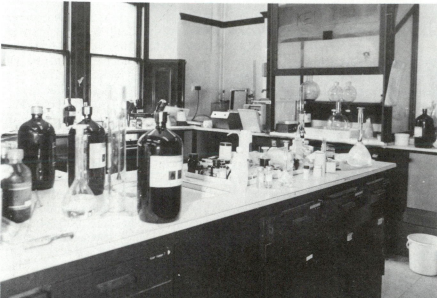

25 (a and b) Part of the department's laboratories at the old accommodation in University Gardens

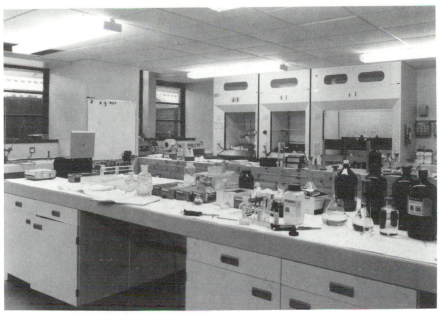

25   (c) Part of the new toxicological laboratory

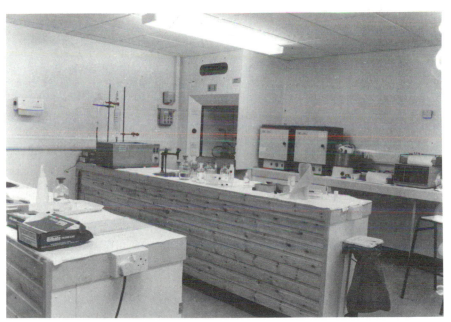

25   (d) Part of the new teaching laboratory (dept of forensic medicine)

requests to act in many parts of Scotland. The following table indicates the flow of work through the department's forensic science laboratory:

CASELOAD IN TOXICOLOGY

YEAR	POST-MORTEMS (drugs/alcohol)	RTO DEFENCE (alcohol)	RTO POLICE (drugs)	GREYHOUNDS (drugs)
1977	598	550	—	567
1978	551	727	—	457
1979	466	737	—	347
1980	439	745	—	414
1981	549	592	—	403
1982	478	688	—	568
1983	462	451	—	501
1984	587	277	—	346
1985	758	363	15	457
1986	938	212	78	405
1987	961	237	39	551

(RTO = Road Traffic Offences.
Source: departmental log books)

There are four technicians working in the laboratories for the three toxicologists, who may be called to give evidence in courts throughout Scotland.

The new department is divided into a series of eight specialised laboratories. The Histology Laboratory prepares specimens for the use of the pathologists: since the younger Glaister's time, the number of days taken to provide the thinly-sliced tissues has been reduced from about ten to two. For certain types of tissue, such as fatty tissue, the freezing microtome provides a very rapid service. The bulk of the laboratory resources, however, are devoted to toxicology, as the ingenuity of the toxicologists has to keep up with the ingenuity of the pharmaceutical industry. Their scientific expertise is constantly devoted not only to detecting the presence of drugs, but determining the quantity as precisely as possible.

All samples undergo preliminary separations in the human tissue laboratory, and the prepared extracts are then distributed to the other laboratories for further treatment and measurement using the various techniques available. In the Instrument Laboratory, all are routinely tested for alcohol by gas chromatography. In the Toxicology Laboratory, the extracts are prepared for analysis by high pressure liquid chromatography and gas liquid chromatography. This equipment detects whether drugs are present, and in what quantities. Before the results can be used as evidence, they must be confirmed by alternative techniques. The Radio Chemistry Laboratory has equipment for radioimmunoassay, which uses the specific antibodies to detect drugs in urine and prepared blood samples, using radioactive material. It identifies not the particular drug, but the group to which it belongs: in combination with other techniques, it is at present the only way of isolating certain commonly-

used drugs such as LSD. The Atomic Absorption Laboratory is for identification and measurement of trace elements.

The most expensive laboratory contains the two mass spectrometers and
their accompanying gas or liquid chromatography units. The original mass
spectrometer, acquired by Arthur Harland, has been complemented by a more
advanced version installed (with some difficulty because of its size), at the
opening of the new department. This equipment can be used, for example, to
identify and measure drugs where other techniques have failed, or when the
sample available is very small. Mass spectrometry is also used in research to
develop more sensitive techniques for finding drugs, and is the most powerful
tool available to the forensic toxicologist.

An important aim of all forensic science laboratories is to reduce to the
minimum the time taken for analysing specimens. In certain cases, such as
serious crimes, delay may seriously impede police investigations. At present,
the usual time taken is about two days, though a particularly urgent request
from the police is dealt with as rapidly as the techniques allow. All the
toxicologists are involved in complex research to identify drugs and poisons
in both humans and animals, and their research is often in co-operation with
colleagues in clinical departments.

Research in forensic pathology tends to arise naturally out of casework.
Subarachnoid haemorrhages were Gilbert Forbes' interest, continued by both
Harland and Watson.[24] These haemorrhages in the back of the neck can occur
spontaneously: the task for forensic pathology was to distinguish spontaneous
haemorrhages from those which resulted from external causes, such as
assault. This might be easy if there were obvious external signs of violence,
but these are not always detected except by careful post-mortem examination.
The research required a case log to be kept on this relatively rare phenomenon.
Amongst other things, Alan Watson is interested in the problem of drowning,
cot deaths, and a syndrome which he calls Hide and Die, in which old people
crawl into most unusual places, such as under floor boards, or into laundry
baskets, before dying.

In describing the research and service work, it should not be forgotten
that all members of the department have responsibility for teaching both
undergraduate and postgraduate students in medicine, law or science. They
also take part in the education of nurses and dentists, and police training
outside the university. In addition to the postgraduate courses set up by
Arthur Harland, there is a new diploma of Forensic Medicine, taught in the
evening and intended for professionals with medico-legal interests, including
doctors, lawyers, social workers and the police. The Regius Professor has
inherited his predecessors' fondness for using the clearest possible slides in
his undergraduate lectures: in a time-honoured response, one or more of the
students will faint.

Both doctors and scientists are often called to appear in court, and the
students still go to observe how they conduct themselves. The medical witnesses often give evidence at considerable length in serious cases: they must,
in the words of the *Ballad*, describe to a jury of laymen in accessible language
'the time and the tool and the manner and place' of death. This requires the

skills in communication recommended to the expert witness since earliest times. In the late nineteenth century it was possible for a regius professor like Harry Rainy to be a good scientist but a bad witness; the modern forensic pathologist cannot afford to follow his example.

The McCluskey report urged that the university departments be represented on a local committee for the general co-ordination of the forensic pathology services. In Glasgow there is now a Forensic Pathology Liaison Committee: it includes the Glasgow and neighbouring procurators fiscal, The Chief Medical Officer to the Strathclyde Police, and representatives of the Crown Office, and the NHS pathologists who work for both Crown and defence.

The daily work of the pathologists also takes them to the city mortuary, which is approaching its own diamond jubilee in 1995. The mortuary stands next to the Judiciary buildings at the foot of Saltmarket, opposite the main entrance to Glasgow Green. It is a landmark in its own right, with the effects of nearly sixty years of exposure to Glasgow's industrial environment clinging to the stone-work and permeating the interior. The structure has changed little since Sillitoe's grand plan.

Under Scots law, the procurator fiscal must inquire into all sudden, suspicious, accidental, unexpected and unexplained deaths: these fall into 22 categories.[25] He does not call for a post-mortem in all cases, but, as in the elder Glaister's time, he will instruct the department to perform this task whenever he sees fit.[26] The fiscal retains his traditional right to call any doctor he pleases, but in practice he usually sends a general summons to the department for one or two pathologists: a rota system with the hospital pathologists is maintained at busy times and weekends. Since 1984, the number of post-mortems conducted by the department has risen rapidly as the pathologists have taken over much of the responsibility for this work in Glasgow and its neighbouring regions. The following table shows this change:

POST-MORTEM STATISTICS

YEAR	TOTAL PMs	OUTSIDE GLASGOW	%	DEFENCE PMs	%
1976	666	135	20	18	2.7
1977	582	112	19	11	2.0
1978	513	124	24	5	1.0
1979	489	137	28	7	1.4
1980	439	74	16	11	2.5
1981	513	86	16	15	3.0
1982	454	78	17	13	2.8
1983	727	108	14	29	4.0
1984	1095	183	16	18	1.6
1985	1005	292	29	12	1.2
1986	1299	342	26	14	1.0
1987	1308	376	28	14	1.0

(source: departmental log books)

The following is an account of procedure at a murder post-mortem.

When the two pathologists arrive at the mortuary the body will have been delivered by the police: relatives or friends who come to identify it wait in a small ante-room, where one of the pathologists joins them to explain why a post-mortem is required, and stays with them until they have identified the body on closed circuit television. Normally, the post-mortem cannot be carried out until the body has been identified. Police officers will be waiting in another ante-room used as an office. Here they give details of the case to the pathologists. The fiscal, or his deputy, in whose domain the body was found, is also present, as are senior members of the CID. The office is surprisingly homely, but despite this, conversation is muted. Some police officers still find attendance at post-mortems an ordeal, in spite of their experience, and Jackie Stirling, the Chief Technician at the City Mortuary, knows how to put them at ease. Twenty-five years service at the mortuary has given him a humane facility for erecting barriers against the task ahead for relatives and policemen alike.

In the post-mortem room, the present ventilation system cannot overcome the redolence of the past. Bodies are brought here directly from the place where they are found: this ranges from a case of sudden death which has been discovered immediately, to the decomposing remains of a long-undiscovered body. This is often a far cry from the work of the hospital pathologist who deals with the recently dead. To the side of the post-mortem room, behind flexible plastic doors, are 51 refrigerated cubicles for the daily toll of sudden or unexplained deaths. Some have occupants of longer duration, usually bodies which, by law, cannot be buried until exhaustive processes have been gone through to identify them; or, occasionally, of bodies where it has proved difficult to ascertain the cause of death.

The body lies on one of the two post-mortem tables. Before the doctors begin the internal examination, they make a careful external examination after reading the police report; they note any marks, abrasions and identifying features. One of the doctors may have visited the scene of the crime, but as the police now make detailed videos, this is less necessary than formerly. Both doctors examine the body, and one takes notes. A police photographer keeps a photographic record which may be used later in evidence. Like their predecessors in the Glasgow department, the doctors sometimes take their own photographs.

The post-mortem of a murder victim is very formal. Certain procedures must be followed before the first doctor actually opens the body. The outcome of the post-mortem will involve both doctors giving evidence before the High Court, therefore detailed preparation is necessary.

If Professor Watson is the first doctor, he is a dramatic figure, completely covered in a protective white rubber gown reaching from neck to ankle, with white rubber boots, and surgical gloves. The second doctor is ready to check all findings, and take detailed notes. Silence is not required, and the Professor makes every effort to inform fiscal and police of his findings as he proceeds. His first action is to take nail clippings, which may contain important forensic evidence, and these are put into plastic bags and labelled. In a normal post-mortem, the body will have been washed by the mortuary attendants, but in a murder case the body is left as it was, and the pathologists wash it themselves. During washing, it is carefully observed for any extraneous substances such as earth, leaves, or paint, which may be kept for analysis. Then the external nature of the injuries is explored. If strangulation is suspected, the doctor looks for small pin-head spots called petechiae in the eyes and eyelids. If there are signs of external injury, the dimensions and outward appearance of any wounds are noted. At this point the doctor is ready to open the body.

Post-mortem methods have not changed greatly since the time of Sir Robert Christison, who, in the mid-nineteenth century, wrote a detailed account of recommended procedure for fiscals to give to their medical examiners. Christison knew that a post-mortem must be painstaking and methodical, and hence best carried out in a regular order. The difference between past and present is not so much in surgical technique, as in how the modern pathologists interpret what they see.

The doctor carefully avoids disturbing external wounds when he makes his incision, which is usually from chin to pubes. The internal examination begins with the chest cavity and abdomen, and the doctor examines the internal organs *in situ*, looking for any obvious causes of death such as the angle of penetration of a knife wound, or the trajectory of a bullet. Internal organs are then removed to a long metal inspection bench, where they are surgically examined to establish the cause of death, but signs of any pre-existing disease are also noted. Samples are taken for histological and toxicological tests. Other parts of the body are then subjected to similar careful scrutiny.

At the end of the autopsy, the Professor discusses with the fiscal how the victim met his death. Afterwards, in the manner of his predecessors, he may find it necessary to go through energetic exercises to demonstrate how the attack occurred. The detective constables carry away productions such as nail clippings to the forensic laboratory. Labels on the bags used for this purpose are signed by the doctor, and will then collect further signatures as they pass through various laboratories. For this reason, Professor Watson signs in a distinctive ink so that he can immediately locate his own signature in court. The post-mortem takes around two hours from first to last.

Normally, after all post-mortems, the pathologist signs the death certificate before he leaves the mortuary. He may later have contact with the relatives, who are anxious to be reassured about the nature of the death, and wishing to have medical terms explained. The modern pathologist does not avoid this task, whereas the experts of the past were usually remote and inaccessible figures. Back in the university, the report is prepared and signed, under the solemn oath so long required of the doctor under Scots law:

'attested on soul and conscience'.

Conclusion: A Layman's View

Where is the doctor of the immediate future to make his acquaintance with the subtleties of the death certificate, the cremation certificate, the certificates of lunacy, the medical report, the problems attendant on malpraxis, the ethical aspects of the conduct of medical practice, and his rights and limitations within the procedural aspects of the law, if not in the class-room of forensic medicine? It is erroneously thought by many that this subject is one almost exclusively directed to the dramas of 'blood and thunder' rather than to law as it is applied to the practice of medicine.[1]

The younger Glaister, who wrote this in 1952, did not always practice what he preached. Although his lectures contained much sound advice on the legal responsibilities of doctors, the students were more interested in accounts of his famous investigations, particularly the Ruxton case. In this book we have tried to follow his example, if not his precept: we have not avoided the 'blood and thunder', but the story of forensic medicine in Glasgow is also intended to show how a service has been created to assist the law in a large city.

Like all medical history, this is an account of specialisation. At the time of the elder Glaister, hardly any aspect of forensic science was outside the range of the medical expert. Since the last war, new scientific techniques have produced paradoxical results: some processes, such as detecting complex drugs in the body, are now a matter only for the professional toxicologist; others, such as a simple check for unlawful levels of alcohol in drivers' blood, have been made accessible to every policeman. The doctor also is now a specialist, trained in pathology: his area is smaller, but he is expected to have a much deeper understanding of it. He must also work as part of a forensic team with his scientific and clinical colleagues.

Although this is a celebratory history of 150 years of forensic medicine in the University of Glasgow, its implications stretch further than the university, or the city. As the McCluskey report recognised, the Scottish universities had long provided expert witnesses for the courts, and the subject became embedded in these institutions in a way which was not common in England. Hence the Scottish universities produced several professors of international reputation in legal medicine—Sir Robert Christison, Sir Henry Littlejohn, Sir Sydney Smith and both the Glaisters. (The Edinburgh professors stood a better chance of receiving a knighthood than the Glasgow professors, for reasons

135

which are best left to speculation). The work of the medical detectives and their successors in forensic pathology and toxicology reflects the growth and development of Scottish society, with all its attendant problems, and the notion of university life as an ivory tower is at its most inappropriate when applied to the duties of the expert witnesses.

As laymen, we have been continually struck by the discrepancy between high public expectations of medical and scientific experts, and the limited public finance devoted to them. Since the late nineteenth century, the experts have been part of popular literature and myth: celebrated in detective stories, biographies, press reports, films and television. Seldom can so many have been so fascinated by so few. The reputations of the great medical detectives, like their famous murder cases, are not readily forgotten. The experts, therefore, are credited with enormous powers, but are not permitted to make mistakes. Given the serious consequences for the liberty of the individual, any departure from the ideal standard results in bitter public criticism.[2]

In spite of this high public reputation, the expert witness, during his years of association with Scottish universities, has not been secure. The first Glasgow Professor of Medical Jurisprudence was imposed on the University from political rather than academic motives, and the future of the chair was often in doubt—a pattern repeated in other Scottish universities from time to time. With the formation of the NHS, and later, with the financial crisis of both the NHS and the universities, the subject seemed in danger throughout the country. Although the crime rate was increasing, and more expert witnesses were needed, neither the universities nor the NHS could finance an expansion which exceeded their own requirements.

Forensic scientists since the war have been largely employed in Home Office laboratories in England and police laboratories in Scotland. The service is tightly stretched, and recent research has shown how intensive work on one major crime can reduce efficiency in dealing simultaneously with lesser crimes.[3] Although there are now relatively large numbers of forensic scientists in post, the annual turnover is small, which reduces its attractiveness as a career choice. Nor does the pressure of work in these laboratories allow much time for research; hence the importance of forensic toxicology and other forensic sciences within the universities.

In the much smaller area of forensic pathology, the career path also remains very uncertain. Training for a medical career takes a long time: the curriculum for those who wish to specialise in pathology after graduating is also very full. Since only a few pathologists will have the chance to specialise further in forensic pathology, it has seemed unecessary to make this a compulsory part of the training. One feature which links the present forensic pathologists to their predecessors in the department, is that very few of them ever *planned* a career in forensic medicine; rather, they have been attracted into it from other branches of pathology because an unexpected opportunity arose. Some have already had experience of medico-legal work arising from their hospital duties, but a young forensic pathologist today will also undertake training after accepting a post in forensic medicine. Skills in pathology may be rapidly adapted: courtroom techniques may be harder to acquire.

By the 1970s the problems of recruitment in forensic medicine were becoming so severe that the Crown agreed to meet the cost of salaries and certain running costs, in order to provide an esssential service for the procurators fiscal. Glasgow, in the most densely populated part of Scotland, has received the largest share of this investment. For the first time in Britain, a number of forensic pathologists in the universities will be supported by the Crown, and this break with tradition provokes certain questions.

The difference between the British and Continental use of expert witnesses has been a perennial subject of debate in the medical profession.[4] In France, for example, the expert witness is called by neither the defence nor the prosecution, but is regarded as the servant of the court, and required to give impartial advice. Under the adversarial system in Britain, the expert is called to speak on behalf of one side, and must be cross-examined to find out whether there is more than one interpretation of the facts.

Since several Scottish medical experts will now be supported by the Crown, it might be argued that they will become a service only to the prosecution, and endanger their reputation for professional impartiality. Those who work only for the prosecution, it is said, become too interested in securing a conviction, and too distant from the interests of the defence—a criticism made (though cautiously) in a recent Home Office report on the Forensic Science service in England.[5]

The arguments against this view, at least in the Scottish context, are as follows: firstly, the new financial arrangements for the forensic pathologists will probably not change the direction of their work to any marked degree. In Glasgow, the two Glaisters rarely acted for the defence, and the number of defence cases in recent years has always been small. On the other hand, Scottish expert witnesses may be precognosed by the defence as well as the prosecution, and their reports are formal pieces of evidence, available to both sides before the trial. The Crown's expert evidence is therefore more available to the defence than under the English system, and the defence may try to establish, in advance of the trial, whether alternative interpretations are possible.

A second persistent tradition in Scottish medico-legal work also runs counter to the popular myth, but also encourages impartial testimony. The Scottish medical witness has never worked single-handed. In all serious cases his findings must be verified by a colleague under the strict rules of corroborative evidence. The formal reports carry two signatures, and if the doctors cannot agree, the procurator fiscal will call in a third opinion. (Only one instance of this has been recalled). The virtues of this double-checking are obvious, but should not be exaggerated. It is unlikely, for example, that a junior doctor will always feel able to contradict the views of a distinguished professor acting as first doctor. On the other hand, a distiguished professor is more likely to remain alert when he knows that his junior is following every move. The 'double-doctor' system also helps to counteract that tendency towards over-confidence which the great medical detectives of the past sometimes recognised in their contemporaries, if not in themselves.[6]

Above all, the doctors supported by the Crown Office will not be located in separate institutions under the direction of government, but in the universities, amongst their clinical and scientific colleagues. They are not employed in working for the Crown only, but have responsibilities in teaching and research. The McCluskey report envisaged that this would prevent intellectual isolation: it might also be seen as a safeguard of impartiality in an imperfect world, as long as the universities themselves remain independent of the state.

Notes

INTRODUCTION pp. 1 to 4.

1   PRO MH 79/387. Trenchard to Lord Atkin, 19 Nov 1934.
2   An excellent guide to the history of forensic medicine is to be found in the introduction to T R Forbes, *Surgeons at the Bailey*, New Haven 1985.
3   Ibid, p. 33.
4   Advocates' Library, Edinburgh: Faculty of Advocates, *Regulations as to Intrants*, 1854.

CHAPTER ONE pp. 5 to 25.

1   GUA Principal Macfarlan's papers, no. 418.
2   Technically, this is still the case, though in practice the Crown patronage office accepts a nomination from the University's appointments committee.
3   GUA 26704, Senate Minutes 89, pp. 209-ll. Also Coutts, *History of the University of Glasgow*, pp. 538-9.
4   Loudon, *Medical Care and the General Practitioner 1750-1850, p. 167 ff.*
5   For a general discussion of the state of forensic medicine in England, see Forbes, *Surgeons at the Bailey.*
6   A discussion of the origins and use of the term 'medical police' can be found in Rosen, *Medical Police* pp. 120-158, and Jordanova, 'Policing public health in France 1780-1815'.
7   G B Risse, *Hospital Life in Enlightenment Scotland*, Cambridge 1986, p. 13.
8   M Robinson (ed), *Concise Scots Dictionary*, Aberdeen 1985, p. 509.
9   J P Frank, *System einer vollständigen medicinischen Polizey*, Mannheim 1778-88.
10   Risse, pp. 274-8; also A Chitnis *The Scottish Enlightenment*, 1976, for a general discussion.
11   See D M Vess, *Medical Revolution in France 1789-1796*, Gainesville 1975.
12   Its history is given in M L Thoinot, 'Histoire de la chaire de médecine légale de la Faculté de Paris', *Annales d'Hygiène Publique et de Médecine Légale* 4th series, 6, 1906, pp. 481-517.
13   EUL, A Duncan, 'A short view of the extent and importance of medical jurisprudence, considered as a branch of education,' 1798.
14   There is a discussion of Duncan's views in White, 'Medical Police,' pp. 408-9. Rosen, op cit p. 152.
15   EUL Edinburgh University Senate minutes vol 2, p. 148.
16   Review of F E Foderé, *Les Lois eclairées par les Sciences Physiques, ou Traité de*

Médecine Légale et d'Hygiène publique, and P A O Mahon, *Médecine légale et Police médicale, Ed.Med.Surg.Jnl.* 1, 1805, p. 331. This review is almost certainly by Duncan himself: it reproduces a large section of his previous 'Memorial'.

17   H W Rumsey, *Essays on State Medicine*, 1856, p. 67.

18   Campbell, 'Some landmarks in the history of arsenic testing', pp. 199-200.

19   *Report to His Majesty by a Royal Commission of Inquiry into the State of the Universities of Scotland*. Evidence, vol 2 (HMSO 1831), p. 130. Also in PP 1831 (cmd 310), xii.

20   Anderson, *Education and Opportunity*, p. 48.

21   Royal Commission 1831, p. 138.

22   Ibid, p. 202.

23   Ibid, p. 146.

24   There is a full account in Anderson, *Education and Opportunity*, ch 2.

25   RCPS Minutes of the Royal College of Physicians and Surgeons of Glasgow 1/1.6 passim.

26   GUA 58434/10.

27   GUL BG33-h.9. Testimonials in favour of Dr James Corkindale, 1832.

28   GUA Senate minutes 89, pp. 64, 69, 72.

29   M W Flinn (ed), *Report on the Sanitary Condition of the Labouring Population of Great Britain by Edwin Chadwick*, Edinburgh 1965, p. 99.

30   R J Morris, *Cholera 1832*, 1976, p. 67.

31   R Cowan, 'Remarks suggested by the Glasgow Bills of Mortality on the morbidity of children', Glasgow, n.d.; 'Statistics of Fever and Small Pox in Glasgow in 1837', Glasgow n.d.; 'Vital Statistics of Glasgow 1838', Glasgow, n.d.

32   Cowan, 'Vital Statistics of Glasgow', p. 13.

33   Anderson, *Education and Opportunity*, p. 50-2.

34   See Loudon, *Medical Care*, p. 298ff.

35   GUA 26704 Senate Minutes 89, p. 138ff.

36   SRO Dalhousie muniments, GD 45/9/9/1.

37   *Lancet* 10 Aug 1839, p. 734.

38   GUA 26704 Senate Minutes 89, p. 211.

39   SRO HH 5/14.

40   Well recounted by House, *Square Mile of Murder*.

41   Many of the public at the time, and most writers subsequently, have thought her lucky in the verdict. See *Notable British Trials: Trial of Madeleine Smith*, pp. 28-9.

42   SRO Dalhousie muniments, GD 45/9/9/1.

43   GUA Senate minutes 89.

44   *Lancet*, 23 Oct, 13 Nov 1941.

45   GUL BG33-h.9. Testimonials on behalf of Robert MacGregor, MD (Glasgow 1841).

46   Wallace Anderson, *Four Chiefs of the Glasgow Royal Infirmary*, pp. 8-9.

47   RCPS Schedule of Rainy's lectures, 1862.

48   For a further discussion see M A Crowther and B M White, 'Medicine, property and the law in Britain 1800-1914', *Historical Journal* (forthcoming).

49   GUA 62848.

50   Christison, *Poisons*, pp. 697, 897.

51   Glaister, *Medical Jurisprudence* (4th edn), p. 800.

52   H Rainy, 'On Reinsch's process for the detection of Arsenic,' *Proceedings of the Glasgow Philosophical Society* 1849.

53   H Rainy, 'On the cooling of dead bodies as indicating the length of time that has elapsed since death', *GMJ* May 1869, pp. 323-30. Rainy's actual equation was

$$\frac{\text{Log D} - \text{Log t}'}{\text{Log r}} = x$$

Where, t = excess of body temperature over atmosphere at first measurement; t−t′ = the excess one hour later; t′+D = excess of temperature of the body at time of death; r = t/t′, x = time elapsed since death.

54   Ibid, p. 330.
55   Ibid, p. 329.
56   For a modern discussion, see L M Al-Alousi and R A Anderson, 'Post-mortem interval by microwave thermography', in Caddy (ed), *Uses of Forensic Science*, pp. 101-15.
57   Information on Scottish probate is published alphabetically in the *Calendar of Confirmations and Inventories* HMSO Edinburgh: information on Rainy in 1876. Probate records tend to underestimate wealth, since they omit certain capital assets.
58   Wellcome MS 3393, notes of A D Maclagen's lectures, 1877.
59   *GMJ* 109, 1928, pp. 85-6.
60   SRO HH 5/42.
61   Two in the Forensic Medicine department at Glasgow; one in the Wellcome Library, taken by J G Douglas Kerr, Wellcome MS 4610; one in the Strathclyde Regional Archives.
62   Taylor, *Principles and Practice of Medical Jurisprudence*, 1865, and later eds.
63   There are many surviving copies of Scottish medical students' lecture notes from various dates in the nineteenth century, in both the Wellcome Library and Edinburgh University library.
64   Wellcome MS 4610; section headings.
65   1883 notes, Glasgow Forensic Medicine dept.
66   GUA Court Minutes 5, pp. 471-2.

CHAPTER TWO pp 26 to 37.

1   Copy of 'The Ballad of John Glaister' in GUA 30615.
2   Correspondence in *GH* 13 March and 18 March 1964.
3   GUA 30633(a) and 30633(e). Glaister, 'History of the Glaister Family in Lanark', unpublished MS (Hereafter Glaister, 'History'.)
4   J. Glaister, *William Smellie and His Contemporaries: a Contribution to the Literature of Midwifery in the Eighteenth Century*, Maclehose, Glasgow 1894.
5   Glaister, 'History'.
6   Glaister, 'History', and GUA 27379 Medical Faculty Minutes 15 June 1877. Glaister therefore at first practised medicine purely on his Edinburgh diplomas.
7   Glaister, 'History'.
8   Glaister often stated that he was first prizeman in forensic medicine and pathology, but not where or when; there is no record of his attending these classes at Glasgow University, but he may have taken the courses either at the Andersonian or GRI.
9   Information from *The Medical Directory* and university calendars.
10   The Medical Act, 49 & 50 Vict. c 48, s. 21.
11   W T Gairdner, *The Physician as Naturalist*, Maclehose, Glasgow 1896. Gairdner stated that there were no university lectures on public health when he was appointed in 1862.
12   We are grateful to Dr Dorothy Porter for alerting us to this episode.

13   Craig, *History of the Royal College of Physicians of Edinburgh*, pp. 530-3. Medical students could take courses offered in the Science Faculty, and then obtain the equivalent of a DPH through the Royal College of Physicians of Edinburgh.
14   *BMJ* 21 June 1890, pp. 1453-4.
15   Glaister, 'Forensic Medicine department', p. 205.
16   'Memorial from Dr. Glaister and others to the General Council of Medical Education and Registration of the United Kingdom,' *Minutes of the General Council* 27 May 1890, pp. 21-37.
17   For details, ibid May-Nov 1890, and Glasgow University Court and Senate minutes for the same period.
18   *Glasgow Herald* 16 Oct 1890, p. 3 shows the degree of local interest.
19   Ibid. The words are those of Professor Leishman, Dean of Medicine, who was also the university's representative on the GMC. Some of the first DPH holders later returned their certificates to the University.
20   These include J Glaister, *Manual of Hygiene for Students and Nurses*, Edinburgh 1897; 'The anti-toxin treatment of diptheria', *Proceedings of the Glasgow Philosophical Society* March 1893; 'Microbes, what they are, and the parts they play', *Sanitary Journal* April 1896;
21   Edinburgh University Calendars, 1897-8.
22   GUA 50570, Court minutes, 21 Jan 1898.
23   GUA 27381, medical faculty minutes, 2 Feb 1898.
24   GUA 50571, Court minutes, 5 May 1898.
25   GUA, Court minutes, 9 Nov 1922.
26   Ibid.
27   GUA Court minutes, 9 Nov 1922.
28   GUA Court minutes, 8 Oct 1931.
29   Glaister, 'Forensic Medicine Department', pp. 201-11.
30   Idem.
31   Ibid, pp. 205-9.
32   Quoted by Sydney Smith, *Mostly Murder*, p. 57.
33   W A Guy and D Ferrier, *Principles of Forensic Medicine* 4th edn 1875.
34   E von Hofmann, *Atlas of Legal Medicine*, ed F Peterson, Philadelphia 1898.
35   J Glaister, *A Textbook of Medical Jurisprudence, Toxicology and Public Health*, 1902. This was the only edition where Glaister conjoined the subjects. For the second edition in 1910 he published the public health section separately as *A Textbook of Public Health*, Livingstone, Edinburgh 1910. Thereafter he published only the textbook on medical jurisprudence and toxicology.
36   Glaister, *Medical Jurisprudence* 4th edn, p. 78. Faulds recognised the unique nature of fingerprints, but did not manage to produce a system of classification as effective as Henry's.
37   D G Browne and A Brock, *Fingerprints: Fifty Years of Scientific Crime Detection*, 1953, chs 2-3.
38   Glaister, *Medical Jurisprudence*, 1st edn p. 75.

CHAPTER THREE pp 38 to 52.

1   The student author is wrong here: the medical report is formally read out in Scottish courts.
2   James Dunlop, 'Notes on acupressure as applied to "street surgery"', *GMJ* new series, 12, 1886-7.

3   *Reports from the Select Committee on Death Certification*, q. 184.
4   *BMJ* 31 Dec 1932, part 2, pp. 1215-6.
5   Fees for Scottish cases are laid down in R J M Buchanan and E W Hope: *Husband's Forensic Medicine, Toxicology and Public Health* 7th edn, 1904, p. 24. Glaister appears to have conformed to these guidelines, from the accounts which survive in GP.
6   Glaister, *Final Diagnosis*, pp. 13-29.
7   Anderson, 'Scottish University Professors', p. 37.
8   Browne and Tullett, *Life of Spilsbury*, p. 198.
9   Grant, *The Thin Blue Line*, p. 101.
10   Glaister, *Medical Jurisprudence* 4th edn, p. 320.
11   Ibid, pp. 319-21.
12   There is an account of this in Grant, *Thin Blue Line*, pp. 72-5.
13   Glaister Jr recounted the story at length in *The People's Journal*, 12 Oct. 1935, p. 28.
14   Ibid, p. 27. See also *GH* 5-6 May 1920.
15   I.e. market crosses, places where official information was traditionally pinned up
16   Example of these conventions in SRO JC 26/1609.
17   E.g. SRO JC 26/1500, (Robert McCully), 4 July 1905.
18   SRO JC 36/49 (John Keen, 1925), p. 193.
19   *GMJ* 7th series, 1933 I, p. 48.
20   Reported in *GH* 29 Dec. 1909 p. 13a; Glaister, *Medical Jurisprudence* 4th edn, p. 213.
21   Glaister, *Medical Jurisprudence* 4th edn, pp. 324-5; details of trial in *Glasgow Citizen*, 25 Feb 1908.
22   The trial is reported in *Notable British Trials: Trial of Oscar Slater*, and there is a popular account in House, *Square Mile of Murder*.
23   Conan Doyle, *The Case of Oscar Slater*. See also W Park, *The Truth about Oscar Slater* (n.d.).
24   *Trial of Oscar Slater*, p. 139.
25   Doyle, *Slater*, p. 69.
26   *Trial of Oscar Slater*, p. lx.
27   Ibid, p. 146.
28   Scottish Home Department, *Criminal Statistics, Scotland 1959*, HMSO Edinburgh, 1960, cmnd 1024 p. 29; J Mack, 'Crime' in Cairncross, *The Scottish Economy*, p. 234.
29   Glaister Jr in *The People's Journal*, 28 Sept 1935, p. 27.
30   *GH* 28 Ap 1919. Glaister's note on cuttings in GP. In *Glaswegian*, 'dugs' = 'dogs'; 'wally' = 'glazed.'
31   Glaister, *Poisoning by Arseniuretted Hydrogen*, chs. xiii-xiv.
32   *The Medical Officer*, 25 June 1910, p. 369.
33   Glaister, *Poisoning by Arseniuretted Hydrogen*, pp. 252-72.
34   Information from Jack House.
35   Roger Smith, 'The boundary between insanity and criminal responsibility in nineteenth-century England', in A Scull (ed), *Madhouses, Mad-doctors and Madmen* Philadelphia 1981, p. 366.
36   The scope of Glaister's activities can be seen in SRO JC/13 (Western Circuit minutes), and JC/14 (Glasgow second court minutes).
37   Glaister, *Medical Jurisprudence* 4th edn, pp. 555-6, 595-7.
38   Glaister, Jr in *The People's Journal* 28 Sept 1935, p. 28.
39   Glaister, 'The future of the race', pp. 40-1.
40   J B Russell, 'Life in one Room', in A K Chalmers (ed), *Public Health Administration in Glasgow*, Glasgow 1904, pp. 189-206.

41   Glaister, 'Future of the Race', p. 42.

CHAPTER FOUR pp 53 to 73.

1   R D Anderson, 'Scottish University Professors', pp. 46-7, shows that professors
     (not all Scottish) were the second largest group of fathers of the Scottish prof-
     essoriat between 1800 and 1929: only the clergy contributed more.
2   Glaister, *Final Diagnosis*, p. 21.
3   Anderson, 'Scottish University Professors', p. 37.
4   A full description is given in Glaister, *Medical Jurisprudence*, 4th edn, pp. 383-91.
5   Smith and Glaister, *Recent Advances*, pp. 99-100.
6   G J F Nuttall, *Blood Immunity and Blood Relationship—the Precipitin Test for Blood*,
     1904.
7   Described, together with a general history of the tests, in William R Smith, 'Blood
     Tests,' *Trans.Med.-Leg. Soc.* viii, 1910-11, pp. 150-62.
8   Correspondence in PRO HO 45/11103.
9   Glaister, *Medical Jurisprudence*, 4th edn pp. 401-2.
10   *GMJ* 1922, 2, pp. 284-5.
11   J Glaister, 'The results of experimental work upon the precipitin or serological
     test for the detection of blood, considered from the medico-legal aspect', unpub-
     lished MD thesis, University of Glasgow, 1925.
12   Smith and Glaister, *Recent Advances*, pp. 119-21.
13   Glaister, *Final Diagnosis*, pp. 44-5. Also copy of medical report in GP.
14   *GET* 31 Jan 1922.
15   *GH* 31 Jan 1922.
16   Copy of medical report in GP.
17   SRO JC 36/49 (John Keen), pp. 283-312.
18   Full transcript in SRO JC 36/49; see also *GET*, 2 Sept 1925.
19   *GH* 22 Jan 1926, p. 4.
20   SRO JC 26/1605.
21   Cf his preparation for the Merrett case, Browne and Tullett, *Bernard Spilsbury*, p.
     333.
22   SRO JC 36/50, p. 269.
23   Ibid, p. 286.
24   SRO JC 36/50, p. 278. Aitchison's question does not appear in the official trial
     transcript, but was quoted in all the newspapers next day: the prosecution
     probably asked for it to be struck from the record. See *GH* 21 Jan 1926, p. 8.
     and *Daily Record* 21 Jan 1926, p. 2.
25   Glaister, *Final Diagnosis*, p. 52.
26   *GH* 22 Jan l926. This is a press paraphrase: SRO JC 36/50 does not include the
     summing-up.
27   *DNB*.
28   Glaister, *Final Diagnosis*, pp. 49-50.
29   SRO JC 36/54 (James M'Kay), p. 204.
30   Ibid, p. 209.
31   Ibid, p. 22.
32   Glaister, *Final Diagnosis*, p. 139.
33   For a useful essay on legal implications of scientific advance, see Brownlie, 'Blood
     and the blood groups'.
34   Smith and Glaister, *Recent Advances*, chs 2-4.
35   J Glaister, 'A study of hairs and wools belonging to the mammalian group of

animals, considered from the medico-legal aspect', unpublished D Sc thesis, University of Glasgow, 1927. *Final Diagnosis*, pp. 41-2.

36 Smith and Glaister, *Recent Advances*, ch. v.

37 J Glaister, *Hairs of mammalia, with a special study of human hair, considered from the medico-legal aspect* (Cairo, 1931).

38 Smith and Glaister, *Recent Advances*, p. 77; SRO JC 26/1615.

39 *Ayrshire Post* 5 Dec 1924. Copy of Glaister's report in GP.

40 GUA, 'Application by John Glaister, Jun. for the appointment of Regius Professor of Forensic Medicine, University of Edinburgh' (1927). It was the custom for such testimonials to be presented as a printed pamphlet.

41 S Smith, *Mostly Murder*, p. 182.

42 There is a full transcript of the trial in *Notable British Trials: Trial of John Donald Merrett*.

43 Attempted suicide was not usually regarded as a crime under Scottish law, but the charge seems to have been made to justify keeping Mrs Merrett in a locked room.

44 Ibid, p. 313.

45 S Smith, *Mostly Murder*, pp. 176-80; Glaister, *Final Diagnosis*, p. 47.

46 GP, J Glaister sr to W Horn, 10 Dec 1926.

47 *Trial of Merrett*, pp. 314-18.

48 Ibid, p. 229.

49 Ibid, p. 228.

50 Ibid, p. 162. This rankled with Smith for years; see *Mostly Murder*, p. 178.

51 *Trial of Merrett*, p. 180.

52 S Smith, *Mostly Murder*, p. 179. Glaister Jr also emphasised the 'worthlessness' of Spilsbury's tests in *Final Diagnosis*, p. 48.

53 Spilsbury referred briefly to his Edinburgh experiments in the trial, see *Trial of Merrett*, p. 233. His report to the defence, not printed in the *Trial*, makes it clear that he did experiment with the murder weapon. Copy in GP, Merrett folder.

54 *Trial of Merrett*, p. 288.

55 GP W Roughead to J Glaister sr, 8 Feb 1928. Merrett folder.

56 Copy of account in GP, Merrett folder.

57 Browne and Tullett, *Spilsbury*, pp. 193-4.

58 SRO JC 36/63, pp. 330, 440.

59 Memo by Roche Lynch, 15 Aug 1923, PRO HO 45/11103.

60 SRO JC 36/63, p. 439.

61 Ibid, p. 324.

62 S Smith, *Forensic Medicine* 3rd edn p. 206.

63 SRO JC 36/63, p. 319.

64 Ibid, p. 417.

65 Ibid, p. 516.

66 J Glaister Jr, *People's Journal* 23 Nov 1935, p. 28, and ibid 16 Nov 1935, p. 28.

67 GP W Guthrie Young to John Glaister, 12 Nov 1931, and Glaister to Young 1 Dec 1931.

68 SRO JC 36/54 (James McKay, 1928), p. 218.

69 Keith Simpson, *Forty Years of Murder: an Autobiography*, 1980, pp. 54-6 describes six such cases from his own observations.

70 *People's Journal*, 21 Sept 1935, p. 12.

71 Smith's account appears in *Mostly Murder*, ch 12.

72 Ibid, p. 242.

73 *GET*, 3 July 1931.

CHAPTER FIVE pp 74 to 92.

1   GUA 'Application and Testimonials by John Glaister, Jun.,...for the appointment of regius professor of Forensic Medicine in the University of Glasgow' (l931).
2   E.g. *GH* 5 Sept 1931, p. 5; *Glasgow Evening News* 5 Sept 1931.
3   GUA Court minutes 8 Oct 1931.
4   Smith and Glaister, *Recent Advances*, ch xi.
5   F Martin, 'The use of ultra violet light in the medico-legal aspect of criminal investigations', unpublished MD thesis, University of Glasgow, 1933.
6   GP 'Science and Criminals' a talk given to the City Business Club of Glasgow 28 April 1932.
7   Mant, 'Milestones in the Development of the British Medicolegal System', p. 162.
8   The elder Glaister also expected this: see GUA Court minutes 8 Oct 1931, p. 256.
9   *Final Diagnosis*, p. 79-80.
10 *GMJ* Jan 1940, p. 55.
11 *Lancet*, 13 Jan 1940, pp. 102-3.
12 Dr Walter Spilg allowed us access to Anderson's notes on anaesthetic deaths at the Victoria Infirmary.
13 SRO JC 36/72 (George Dollin), p. 64.
14 Ibid, p. 281.
15 Ibid, pp. 284-7.
16 Ibid, p. 334.
17 Ibid, p. 370.
18 Glaister, *Final Diagnosis*, p. 80. This is a very guarded account, and we have not been able to locate the cases which caused the argument. It is possible that Glaister was not actually appearing for the defence, but giving full advice to defence counsel when they precognosed him.
19 Glaister, *Medical Jurisprudence*, 7th edn 1942, pp. 17-18.
20 According to SRO JC 15 series for this period. For an account of the gangs see Cockerill, *Sillitoe*, pp. 141ff.
21 Smith gives a full account of this case in *Mostly Murder*, ch 14.
22 There is a copy of his report in GP.
23 *Scotsman*, 21 July 1934.
24 S Smith, *Mostly Murder*, pp. 271-2.
25 GUA 50562 GU Court camera minutebook 12, 3 March 1937, p438.
26 Ambage Ph D, 'The origins and development of the Home Office forensic science service', chs 3-4.
27 PRO MH 79/387 gives some of the details. Cf also Ambage, op cit p. 72. Glaister's own memory in *Final Diagnosis*, that he was only offered Hendon after the Ruxton case, is wrong.
28 Ibid, pp. 70-2.
29 Grant, *Thin Blue Line*, p. 101.
30 Cockerill, *Sillitoe*, pp. 85-6.
31 Glasgow's forensic science service was not removed from the direct control of the police until 1965. Grant, *Thin Blue Line*, p. 104.
32 *ARCCG*, 1934, p. 21.
33 SRA DTC 14.2.21/1399. Cockerill, *Sillitoe*, p. 108.
34 SRA DTT 14.2.(23).
35 *GH* 15 April 1933, p. 7.
36 SRA Minutes of Glasgow Corporation Cl.3.94 p. 1003; Cl.3.95 p. 1533; Cl.3.96, p. 1269.

37   'Decline of the English Murder,' reprinted in *Collected Essays, Journalism and Letters of George Orwell*, vol 4, Penguin 1968, p. 126.
38   Ruxton's diary jottings were obtained by the press, and there is a transcript in GP, in which this insult occurs frequently.
39   Smith's and Glaister's.
40   Smith mentions the younger Glaister four times, all in connection with the Ruxton case: Glaister mentions Smith once, in connection with Cairo.
41   Grant, *Thin Blue Line*, pp. 102-3.
42   Depositions at Johnstonebridge police station 28 Oct 1935. Transcript in GP.
43   Glaister and Brash, *Ruxton Case*, chs III, VIII.
44   Glaister, *Final Diagnosis*, pp. 111-2.
45   *Notable British Trials: Trial of Buck Ruxton*, p. 146.
46   Glaister and Brash, *Ruxton Case*, p. 214.
47   *Trial of Ruxton*, p. 165.
48   Ibid, p. 154.
49   *Sunday Dispatch*, 24 Nov 1935.

CHAPTER SIX pp 93 to 113.

1   These, and subsequent figures, are compiled from *ARCCG* which, until the outbreak of war, also give details of each murder and culpable homicide.
2   Ibid. The Chief Constable's reports do not include detailed statistics for 1942 and 1943.
3   Walls, 'Forensic Science Service in Great Britain', p. 278. *ARCCG* 1949, p. 12.
4   This relationship with the police is sometimes criticised, e.g. Lord Morton, 'Forensic medicine—an independent science?' in Caddy, *Uses of the Forensic Sciences*, pp. 89-92.
5   *GH* 30 Jan 1842. Glaister's reports from GP
6   Glaister's report in GP.
7   *Evening Citizen* 14 Dec 1946, p. 1.
8   Glaister and police reports in GP. *GET* 27 March 1946, p. 1.
9   Dawood Matta, 'A clinical investigation of the blood groups and their medico-legal application', unpublished Ph D thesis, University of Glasgow, 1937.
10   GUA 51232 a & b.
11   GUA GU Court Minutes, Finance Committee 1944-5, p. 110.
12   Walls, 'Forensic science service in Great Britain' for short account.
13   Mant, 'Forensic Medicine: what is its future?' p. 17.
14   A K Mant, 'A Survey of forensic pathology in England since 1945', *Jnl.Forensic Sci.Soc.* 13 (1973), p. 22.
15   Glaister, 'Whither Forensic Medicine?' p. 475.
16   Glaister refers to it in these terms, although obliquely, in op cit p. 475.
17   Ministry of Health/Department of Health for Scotland, *Report of the inter-departmental Committee on Medical Schools* (HMSO 1944), p. 161.
18   For events in this period see Glaister, 'Whither Forensic Medicine?' p. 473.
19   Ibid, pp. 474-5.
20   Ibid, p. 473.
21   *GH* 16 Jan 1947, p. 6. See also SRA Cl-3-114, p. 1492.
22   GUA Court Minutes 1947/8, p. 4.
23   Lenihan, 'Adventures in activation analysis', p. 125.
24   Ibid, p. 127.
25   H Smith, 'The interpretation of the arsenic content of human hair', *Jnl. Forensic Science Soc.* 4, 1964, pp. 192-9.

26 W A Dewar and J M A Lenihan, 'A Case of chronic arsenical poisoning', *Scot.Med.Jnl.* 1, 1956, pp. 236-7.
27 H Smith, S Forshufvud and A Wassen, 'Arsenic content of Napoleon I's hair probably taken immediately after his death', *Nature* 192, 1961, pp. 103-5; and 'Distribution of arsenic in Napoleon's hair', ibid, 194, 1962, pp. 725-6.
28 S Forshufvud, H Smith and A Wassen, 'Napoleon's illness 1816-21 in the light of activation analyses of hairs from various dates', *Archiv fur Toxikologie* 20, 1964, pp. 210-19.
29 Lenihan, 'Adventures in activation analysis', pp. 129-31: J M A Lenihan, A C D Leslie, H Smith, 'Mercury in the Hair of Robert Burns', *Lancet* 1971, 2, p. 1030; information from Prof J Lenihan.
30 J M A Lenihan, 'The application of nuclear physics to the study of historical problems', *Proceedings and Transactions of the Rhodesia Scientific Association* 50, 1964.
31 G S Nixon and H Smith, 'Hazard of mercy poisoning in the dental surgery', *Jnl. of Oral Therapeutics and Pharmacology* 1, 1965, pp. 512-4.
32 GUA Court Minutes 26 May 1955, p. 289.
33 Glaister describes the case in *Final Diagnosis*, pp. 144-9.
34 Glaister's reports, copies of post-mortem and police evidence in GP. *Evening Citizen* 10 Nov 1950, p. 1.
35 GP, Glaister's accounts.
36 Dr Andrew Allison jr remembered this.
37 *BMJ* 1927, i, supplement p. 53. Keith Simpson, *Forensic Medicine* (5th edn 1964), p. 326.
38 Rentoul, Smith, Beavers, 'Some observations on the effects of the consumption of alcohol', p. 2.
39 Brownlie, 'Blood and the blood groups', p. 130.
40 *Cases Decided in the Court of Session* 1958, pp. 450.
41 The case is also discussed in Brownlie, 'Blood and the blood groups', pp. 170-2;
42 Mason, *Forensic Medicine for Lawyers*, p. 185n.
43 *Daily Herald*, 11 Sept 1962.
44 *Scottish Daily Express*, 12 Sept 1968.
45 Smith, 'History and development of forensic medicine'. p. 606.

CHAPTER SEVEN pp 114 to 134.

1 GUA 55142, letter from the Dean of Medicine 16 March 1962.
2 GUA 55142, 2 May 1962.
3 GUA 55142, 28 March 1963.
4 GUA 55142 File on the appointment of Gilbert Forbes.
5 R D Teare, 'Facilities for forensic pathological investigation,' *Med.Sci.Law* 1, 1960-1, p. 288.
6 Glaister, *Final Diagnosis*, p. 142.
7 G Forbes, 'The organisation, staffing and equipment of an institute of forensic medicine', in Simpson (ed), *Modern Trends in Forensic Medicine* 2, p. 27.
8 Havard, *Detection of Secret Homicide*, especially ch 14.
9 *Report of the Committee on Death Certification and Coroners* PP 1971-2 cmd 4810, xxi p. 400. It was argued, however, that in the majority of cases the discrepancy between death certificate and post-mortem report was not significant.
10 Ibid, p. 476. It was, in any case, difficult to arrange autopsies in the thinly populated areas of Scotland.

11   We will term it the McCluskey report for convenience. For provenance, see bibliography.

12   McCluskey report, para 91.

13   Ibid, para 99.

14   Allan and Normand, 'Forensic pathology services in Scotland'. (unpublished)

15   This, and other technical developments are described in J S Oliver, 'Forensic Toxicology', in Mason, *Forensic Medicine for Lawyers*.

16   Numerous publications resulted from this project; a full summary of its scope is given in R A Anderson, A A Watson and W A Harland, 'Fire deaths in the Glasgow area I: General considerations and pathology', *Med.Sci.Law* 21, 1981, pp. 175-83.

17   A A Watson and J S Oliver, 'Some social implications of fire-related deaths,' *International microfilm Journal of Legal Medicine* 11, 1976, article 255.

18   R A Anderson, A A Watson and W A Harland, 'Fire deaths in the Glasgow area II: the role of Carbon monoxide', Ibid, 21, 1981, pp. 288-94: Anderson and Harland, 'Fire deaths in Glasgow III: the role of hydrogen cyanide', Ibid, 22, 1982, pp. 35-40.

19   Harland's views are set out in W A Harland, 'Should Forensic Medicine be allowed to die?', *Scot.Med.Jnl.* 22, 1977, pp. 193-4.

20   'Report of the Department of Forensic Medicine and Science 1974-1982', GUL College Collection.

21   This marks the point where the traditional 40 lectures were reduced to 20, at the beginning of 1976.

22   Information from Professor Harland and the GP concerned.

23   Allan and Normand, 'Forensic pathology services in Scotland'.

24   E.g. W A Harland, J F Pitts, A A Watson, 'Subarachnoid haemorrhage due to upper cervical trauma', *Jnl.Clin. Pathol.* 36, 1983, pp. 1335-41.

25   Carmichael, *Sudden Deaths*, pp. 4-5.

26   The use of the masculine pronoun disguises the fact that an increasing number of fiscals are women.

CONCLUSION pp 135 to 138.

1   J Glaister, 'Whither Forensic Medicine?' *BMJ* 30 Aug. 1952, p. 474.

2   A famous example is the fate of Dr Clift, an English forensic scientist who gave evidence in a Scottish trial. See Alistair R Brownlie, 'Expert evidence in the light of *Preece v. H.M.Advocate*', *Med.Sci.Law* 22, 1982.

3   *The Effectiveness of the Forensic Science Service*, Home Office Research Study 92, HMSO 1987.

4   E.g. William Cummin, 'Practice of forensic medicine, as conducted in this and other countries', *London Medical Gazette* 13, 1834; T Gray, 'The medico-legal expert in France', *Lancet* 1929, pp. 22-4; T Lund, 'Expert evidence', *Med.Sci.Law* 3, 1962-3

5   *The Effectiveness of the Forensic Science Service*, p. 45.

6   The unfortunate Spilsbury was described thus by Smith, *Mostly Murder*, p. 179ff, 192; and Simpson p. 93; Simpson also accuses Camps of growing megalomania, p. 231-2.

Select Bibliography

1 PRIMARY SOURCES

i   JC series in the Scottish Record Office. This is the major source for pre-cognitions and trial material.

ii Glasgow University Archives, which include minutes of Court and Senate, and some papers relating to the Glaisters and individual members of staff.

iii Papers of John Glaister jr, abbreviated as GP. These include files of press cuttings, carbon copies of post-mortem reports (which are also in the SRO), and some personal material. These are in the keeping of Dr David McLay, Chief Medical Officer of the Strathclyde Police, and were made available to us through his courtesy.

iv Manuscripts of student lecture notes from various dates in the 19th century. The best collections are in the Library of the University of Edinburgh and the Wellcome Library in London. Some have also been privately loaned, as indicated in footnotes.

v   Strathclyde Regional Archives: Corporation Minutes and Reports of the Chief Constable of Glasgow/Strathclyde.

2 OFFICIAL PAPERS

Report to His Majesty by a Royal Commission of Inquiry into the State of the Universities of Scotland, 1831 xii cmd 310.

Evidence, oral and documentary, taken and received by the Comissioners for Visiting the Universities of Scotland 1837 xxxvi cmd 93.

General Report of the Commissioners under the Universities (Scotland) Act 1858 1863 xvi cmd 3174.

Report of the Committee on Death Certification and Coroners 1971-2 xxi cmd 4810. (Brodick Committee).

Ministry of Health/Department of Health for Scotland, *Report of the inter-departmental Committee on Medical Schools*, HMSO 1944 (Goodenough Report)

Scottish Home and Health Department and Crown Office, 'Forensic Pathology Services in Scotland.' (McCluskey-Bowen Report). The report, presented in 1975, was not printed: a typescript copy was made available by courtesy of the Crown Office.

3 OTHER UNPUBLISHED MATERIAL

Allan, J Douglas, and Normand, Andrew C,' 'Forensic Pathology Services in Scotland,' paper presented at the 10th triennial meeting of the international association of forensic sciences, Oxford 1984.

150

Ambage, Norman, 'The origins and development of the Home Office forensic science service 1931-1967,' Ph D, University of Lancaster, 1987.

Phillipson, Nicholas, 'The Scottish Whigs and the Reform of the Court of Session 1785-1830,' Ph D, Cambridge 1967.

4   PRINTED BOOKS AND PAMPHLETS

(The place of publication is London, unless otherwise stated)

Alison, Archibald, *Principles of the Criminal Law of Scotland*, Blackwood, Edinburgh 1832

——*Practice of the Criminal Law of Scotland*, Blackwood, Edinburgh 1833

Anderson, J Wallace, *Four Chiefs of the Glasgow Royal Infirmary*, McKinlay, Glasgow 1916

Anderson, Robert D, *Education and Opportunity in Victorian Scotland*, OUP, Oxford 1983

Baker, J L *An Introduction to English Legal History*, Butterworth 1979

Barclay, Hugh, *Criminal Law in Scotland: an Address*, Murray, Glasgow 1862

Brittain, R P *Bibliography of Medico-Legal Works in English*, Sweet & Maxwell, Oxford 1962

Browne, Douglas G and Tullett, E V, *Bernard Spilsbury, His Life and Cases*, Harrap 1951

Browne, G Lathom and Stewart, C G, '*Reports of Trials for Murder by Poison by Prussic Acid, Strychnia, Antimony. Arsenic and Aconitis*, Stevens 1883

Caddy, Brian (ed), *Uses of the Forensic Sciences: the Proceedings of the conference held in Glasgow in April 1986*, Scottish Academic Press, Edinburgh 1987

Cairncross, A K (ed), *The Scottish Economy*, CUP, Cambridge 1954

Carmichael, Ian H B, *Sudden Deaths and Fatal Accident Inquiries: Scots Law and Practice*, W Green, Edinburgh 1986

Christison, Robert, *A Treatise on Poisons* (4th edn), A & C Black, Edinburgh 1855

——*The Life of Sir Robert Christison, Bart. Edited by his Sons* 2v, Blackwood, Edinburgh 1885

Cockburn, Henry, *Memorials of His Time* ed Karl F C Miller, University of Chicago Press 1974

Cockerill, A W, *Sir Percy Sillitoe*, W H Allen 1975

Comrie, John D, *History of Scottish Medicine* 2 vols, Wellcome 1932

Coutts, J, *History of the University of Glasgow 1851-1909*, Maclehose, Glasgow 1909

Craig, W S, *History of the Royal College of Physicians of Edinburgh*, Blackwell, Edinburgh 1976

Doyle, Sir Arthur Conan, *The Case of Oscar Slater*, 1914

Forbes, Thomas Rogers, *Surgeons at the Bailey: English Forensic Medicine to 1878*, Yale University Press 1985

Gatrell, V A C, Lenman, Bruce, and Parker, Geoffrey, *Crime and the Law: the Social History of Crime in Western Europe since 1500*, Europa 1980

Glaister, John sr, *Textbook of Medical Jurisprudence, Toxicology and Public Health*, Livingstone, Edinburgh 1902

——*Poisoning by Arseniuretted Hydrogen or Hydrogen Arsenide*, Livingstone, Edinburgh 1908

——*Textbook of Public Health* (2nd edn) 1910

——*A Textbook of Medical Jurisprudence and Toxicology*, (4th edn) Livingstone, Edinburgh 1921

Glaister, John jr, *A Study of Hairs and Wools Belonging to the Mammalian Group of Animals, considered from the Medico-legal Aspect*, Misr Press, Cairo 1931.

——*Medical Jurisprudence and Toxicology* (9th edn), Livingstone, Edinburgh 1950.

——*Final Diagnosis*, Huchinson 1964

Glaister, John jr, and Brash, James Couper, *Medico-Legal Aspects of the Ruxton Case*, Livingstone, Edinburgh 1937

Gordon, Gerald E, *The Criminal Law of Scotland*, Green, Edinburgh 1967

Grant, Douglas, *The Thin Blue Line: the Story of the City of Glasgow Police*, John Long 1973

Hamilton, David N H, *The Healers. A History of Medicine in Scotland*, Canongate, Edinburgh 1981

Havard, J D J, *The Detection of Secret Homicide: a study of the medico-legal system of investigation of sudden and unexplained deaths*, Macmillan 1960

Holdsworth, W S, *A History of English Law*, 9 vols Methuen

House, Jack, *Square Mile of Murder*, Edinburgh 1961

Loudon, I, *Medical Care and the General Practitioner 1750-1850*, OUP, Oxford 1986

Mason, John Kenyon, *Forensic Medicine for Lawyers* (2nd edn), Butterworths 1983

Nemec, Jaroslav, *International Bibliography of the History of Legal Medicine*, Washington, US Dept of Health and Welfare, n.d.

Notable British Trials series, Hodge, Edinburgh

   Trial of Oscar Slater, (ed Roughead, William), 1910

   Trial of Madeleine Smith (ed Tennyson Jesse, F), 1927

   Trial of John Donald Merrett, (ed Roughead, William) 1929

   Trial of Buck Ruxton (ed Blundell, E H, and Haswell, G), 1937

Omond, George W T, *The Lord Advocates of Scotland: From the Close of the Fifteenth century to the Passing of the Reform Bill* II, David Douglas, Edinburgh 1883

Radzinowicz, Leon, *A History of English Criminal Law and its Administration from 1750*, I Stevens 1948

Rosen, George, *From Medical Police to Social Medicine*, NY 1974

Sheehan, A V, *Criminal Procedure in Scotland and France*, HMSO, Edinburgh 1975

Simpson, Cedric Keith (ed), *Modern Trends in Forensic Medicine* no. 2, Butterworths 1967

——*Forty Years of Murder: an Autobiography*, Grafton 1978

Smith, John Gordon, *The Principles of Forensic Medicine, systematically arranged, and applied to British Practice*, Underwood 1821

Smith, Sydney, *Forensic Medicine: A Textbook for Students and Practitioners*, (3rd edn), J & A Churchill 1931

   Mostly Murder, Panther 1954

Smith, Sydney and Glaister, John jr, *Recent Advances in Forensic Medicine*, J & A Churchill 1931.

[Syme, James], *Illustrations of Medical Evidence and trial by Jury in Scotland*, Sutherland & Knox, Edinburgh 1855

Taylor, Alfred Swaine, *The Principles and practice of Medical Jurisprudence*, Churchill 1865

Watson, Alexander, *Medico-Legal Treatise on Homicide by External Violence*, MacLachlan, Stewart & Co, Edinburgh 1842

5 ARTICLES

Anderson, Robert D, 'Scottish University Professors, 1800-1939: profile of an elite,' *Scottish Economic & Social History* 7, 1987

Brownlie, Alistair R, 'Blood and the blood groups: a developing field for expert evidence,' *Jnl. Forensic Sci.Soc.* 5, 1965

   'Expert evidence in the light of *Preece v. H.M.Advocate*,' *Med.Sci.Law* 22, 1982

Campbell, W A, 'Some landmarks in the history of arsenic testing,' *Chemistry in Britain* 1, 1965

Gardner, J C, 'Inquiry into sudden deaths in England and Scotland,' *Juridical Review* 58, 1946

Glaister, John sr, 'Death certification and registration in Scotland, its present defects and a proposed remedy,' *GMJ* Oct. 1893
 'The law of infanticide, a plea for its revision,' *EMJ* July 1895
 'The future of the race: a study in present day aspects of social bionomics,' *Proceedings of the Royal Philosophical Society of Glasgow* 43, 1912
 'The teaching of Forensic Medicine,' *BMJ* 10 Sept 1927
 'Forensic Medicine Department, University of Glasgow,' in *Methods and Problems of Medical Education*, 9th series, Rockefeller Foundation, NY 1928

Glaister, John jr, 'Whither Forensic Medicine?' *BMJ* 30 Aug 1952

Harland, Walter Arthur, 'Should forensic medicine be allowed to die?' *Scottish Medical Journal* 22, July 1977

Johnson, C H, 'Education and Training of Police Surgeons,' *Med.Sci.Law* 1, 1960-1

Jordanova, Ludmilla J, 'Policing public health in France 1780-1815,' in T Ogawa (ed) *Public Health*, Proceedings of the 5th International symposium on the comparative history of medicine—East and West. Tokyo 1981

Lenihan, John M A, 'Activation analysis in the contemporary world: questions and answers,' in *Modern Trends in Activation Analysis*, National Bureau of Standards Special Publication 312, i, 1969
 'Adventures in Activation Analysis, 1953-1978,' *Jnl. Radioanalytical Chemistry* 48, 1979

Lund, Thomas, 'Expert evidence,' *Med.Sci.Law* 3, 1962-3

Maclagan, Douglas, 'Forensic medicine from a Scotch point of view,' *BMJ* 17 Aug 1878

Mant, A Keith, 'A survey of forensic pathology in England since 1945,' *Jnl.Forensic Sci.Soc.* 13, 1973
 'Milestones in the Development of the British medico-legal system,' *Med.Sci.Law* 17, 1977
 'Forensic Medicine: what is its Future?' *American Jnl. of Forensic Medicine and Pathology* 7, 1986
 'Changes in the practice of forensic pathology 1950-85,' *Med.Sci.Law* 26, 1986

Nicholls, L C, 'The development of forensic science,' *Medico-Legal J.* 27 1959

Rainy, Harry, 'On Reinsch's process for the detection of arsenic,' *Proceedings of the Glasgow Philosophical Society* 1849
 'On the cooling of dead bodies as indicating the length of time that has elapsed since death,' *GMJ* new series, 1, May 1869

Rentoul, Edgar; Smith, Hamilton; Beavers, Richard, 'Some observations on the effects of the consumption of alcohol and its relation to road traffic,' *Jnl.Forensic Sci.Soc.* 2, 1962

Simpson, Cedric Keith, 'The development of forensic medicine,' *Guy's Hospital Gazette* 78, 1964

Smith, Sydney, 'The history and development of forensic medicine,' *BMJ* 24 March 1951

Teare, R D, 'Facilities for forensic pathological investigation,' *Med.Sci.Law* 1, 1960-1

Thomas, F, 'Milestones in forensic science,' *Jnl.Forensic Sci.Soc.* 19, 1974

Walls, H J, 'The forensic science service in Great Britain: a short history,' *Jnl.Forensic Science Soc.* 16, 1976

White, Brenda M, 'Medical police. Politics and Police; the fate of John Roberton,' *Med.Hist.* 27 1983

Index

To avoid confusion and duplication the term forensic medicine is used to include medical jurisprudence, forensic medicine, and forensic science.

Abbreviations: JG I = John Glaister Senior
                      JG II = John Glaister Junior
                      DFM = Glasgow University Department of Forensic Medicine and
                              Science